Prescribing Adult Intravenous Nutrition

Prescribing Adult Intravenous Nutrition

Peter David Austin

BPharm MRPharmS DipClinPharm MSc (PTQA)
  Supplementary Prescriber (UK)

Senior Pharmacist Nutrition Support Team,
Pharmacy Department, Southampton General Hospital,
Southampton, UK

Mike Stroud

BSc MBBS MD DSc MRCP (UK) FRCP (London & Edinburgh)

Consultant Gastroenterologist and Senior Lecturer in Medicine and
  Nutrition
The Institute of Human Nutrition,
Southampton General Hospital,
Southampton, UK

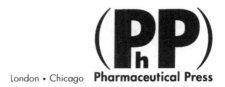

London • Chicago **Pharmaceutical Press**

Published by the Pharmaceutical Press

1 Lambeth High Street, London SE1 7JN, UK
University City Science Center, Suite 5E, 3624 Market Street,
Philadelphia, PA 19104, USA

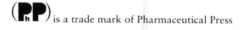 is a trade mark of Pharmaceutical Press

Pharmaceutical Press is the publishing organisation of the
Royal Pharmaceutical Society

First published 2007

Index provided by Indexing Specialist, Hove, East Sussex, UK
Typeset by Type Study, Scarborough, North Yorkshire, UK
Printed and bound by CPI Group (UK) Ltd, Croydon, CR0 4YY

ISBN 978 0 85369 658 2

A catalogue record for this book is available from the British Library

To all who care about patient nutrition

Contents

Preface   xiii
Acknowledgements   xv
About the authors   xvii
Abbreviations   xix

1   The importance of nutrition support   1
Why worry about nutrition?   1
The effects of malnutrition   2
Who needs nutrition support?   3
Ethical issues in nutrition support   4
References   5

2   Oral and enteral tube support   7
Oral nutrition support   7
Enteral tube feeding (ETF)   10
Types of enteral feed   12
Conclusion   18
References   18

3   Intravenous support   19
Who needs intravenous nutrition?   19
Venous access   28
Complications of intravenous nutrition   32
Does intravenous nutrition work?   32
References   33

4   Clinical history and examination   35
Introduction   35
Patient details and reason for referral   36
Taking a clinical history   37
Reviewing laboratory results   43
Clinical examination   45
Reviewing fluid balance, fluid prescription and nutrient intake
    charts   48
Conclusion   51

5   **Review of prescription charts**   53
          Introduction   53
          Information on other medical conditions   54
          Drugs interfering with gut function   54
          Gastrointestinal tolerance and best-prescribed routes for all
              drugs   55
          Interactions between intravenous drugs and intravenous
              nutrition   57
          Avoiding problems from drugs given via enteral feeding
              tubes   58
          Prescribing nutrition support products and drugs related to
              intravenous nutrition   59
          The effects of all prescribed drugs on potential intravenous
              nutrition regimens   60
          Allergies, sensitivities and restrictions   60
          Specialist prescription charts   60
          Administration of intravenous drugs   61
          References   61

6   **Decisions on intravenous nutrition**   63
          Introduction   63
          Intravenous nutrition required   63
          No intravenous nutrition required   64
          Documenting your decisions   65
          Conclusion   69
          References   70

7   **Fluid and macronutrient requirements**   71
          Introduction   71
          Fluid requirements   71
          Levels of energy provision   75
          Nitrogen for non-energy purposes   83
          Balancing macronutrient provision   85
          Starting intravenous nutrition feeding   86
          Continuing intravenous nutrition feeding   87
          Specialised macronutrients   89
          References   92

8   **Electrolytes in intravenous nutrition**   95
          Introduction   95
          Balance and imbalance   95
          Interpreting biochemical results   98
          Electrolyte monitoring   101
          Consequences of electrolyte imbalance   102

Individual electrolyte considerations   105
Standard electrolyte prescribing   115
Prescribing with risk of refeeding syndrome   117
Correcting severe specific electrolyte abnormalities   118
Practical issues in electrolyte prescribing   121
References   123

9   Micronutrients   125
Introduction   125
Causes and consequences of micronutrient depletion   126
Consequences of micronutrient depletion   129
Measuring micronutrient status   137
Principles and practice of micronutrient prescribing   138
Practical aspects of micronutrient prescribing   143
References   144

10   Prescribing for patients with specific problems   147
Introduction   147
Renal compromise   147
Liver disease   150
Pancreatitis, pancreatic insufficiency and diabetes   152
Cardiac failure   154
Respiratory failure   154
Short-bowel syndrome and high-output gastrointestinal
    fistulae   155
References   160

11   Regimen choice   161
Introduction   161
Precompounded and sterilised triple-chamber bags   161
Choosing a regimen   162
Designing your own regimen   168
Regimen compromise   174
Where to prescribe your regimen   178

12   Complications of intravenous nutrition   179
Introduction   179
Complications of intravenous catheter insertion   179
Infective complications from intravenous nutrition   182
Occlusive catheter complications   185
Thrombophlebitis   189
Metabolic complications of intravenous nutrition   195
Conclusions   199
References   199

13   Monitoring   201
Introduction   201
Clinical monitoring of intravenous nutrition patients   201
Laboratory monitoring in the acute setting   207
Monitoring issues in long-term IVN patients   210
References   212

14   Organising nutrition support   213
Introduction   213
Organisation of local nutrition services   213
Different types of nutrition support team   214
The structure of an active nutrition support team   216
Roles within an active nutrition support team   217
Data collection, management and review   222
Funding opportunities for nutrition support teams   229
References   231

15   Technical Services   233
Introduction   233
Why compound intravenous nutrition regimens in Technical
   Services?   233
Final bag release   236
Technical Services' workload   238
Contracting and local component stocks   240
Technical Services licensing (UK)   243
References   244

16   On the ward   245
Introduction   245
Timing of intravenous nutrition administration   245
Starting an intravenous nutrition bag   245
Stopping intravenous nutrition   250
References   253

Final note   255

Appendix 1   Stability   257
Introduction   257
Physical stability   257
Chemical stability   259
Assessing the stability of intravenous nutrition regimens   260
Microbiological stability   263
References   270

Appendix 2   Salts and pharmaceutical calculations   271
Introduction   271
Salts   271
Units of concentration and measurement   273
Pharmaceutical calculations   276
References   280

Appendix 3   Micronutrient preparations   281
Introduction   281
Potential micronutrient products   282
Typical specific micronutrient supplementation   286
References   286

**Appendix 4   High-sodium drinks and feeds for
short-bowel syndrome**   287
Introduction   287
Formulae examples for high-sodium-with-glucose powders to be
    made into a solution with water   287
Adding sodium to enteral feeds   290
References   291

Index   293

The colour plate section is between pages 172 and 173

Preface

Intravenous nutrition (IVN), also known as parenteral nutrition (PN), involves the administration of nutrients, electrolytes, minerals and fluid directly into patients' veins. It is used in patients whose gastrointestinal absorption of food and/or fluids is inadequate, unsafe or inaccessible. Infusing a mixture of nutrients and fluid, however, is not without risk. The placement of an intravenous catheter into a large central vein can cause traumatic damage, and the infusion of what is effectively an ideal bacterial culture medium can easily lead to infection, particularly catheter-related sepsis. The presence of a catheter in the vein can also cause thrombosis with the potential for dislodgement of the clot and pulmonary embolus. If IVN is given into smaller peripheral veins, it can lead to thrombophlebitis. Finally, whatever the route of administration, the provision of artificial nutrition to patients who are very ill and/or malnourished can easily cause metabolic disturbance.

Minimising the risks of IVN and knowing how to treat any complications that do occur require skill. Decisions on its use must therefore be made by individuals who understand both the benefits and the problems of the technique and, having decided that it is really necessary, they should prescribe with logic and care. The use of IVN by individuals lacking such expertise causes complications, adds to the expense and can be a direct threat to health, whereas, used properly, IVN can be life-saving. The aim of this book is to ensure best usage while minimising risks and costs.

The book focuses on the prescribing process of intravenous nutrition support but starts by describing why nutritional care in general is so important. It then briefly discusses patients who might need oral or enteral feeding as well as those who need IVN before it moves on to what should be given, what can go wrong and how to deal with any IVN-related problems. Finally, it covers the organisational aspects of nutritional care, emphasising that doctors, nurses, dietitians and pharmacists must work together in multidisciplinary nutrition support teams to make the right decisions on the wards. Meanwhile, behind the scenes, pharmacists and pharmacy Technical Services units must also undertake vital roles to ensure patient safety and cost-effectiveness.

Peter Austin
Mike Stroud
December 2006

Acknowledgements

Most of the principles and practices outlined in this book were developed over a number of years by members of the Southampton NHS Trust Nutrition Support Team and Institute of Human Nutrition under the leadership of Professor Alan Jackson. Both of us are very grateful for the education in nutritional care that we have received through working with those individuals, an education that this book attempts to pass on to others.

About the authors

Peter Austin graduated from the University of Bath in 1998. After this, he worked as a pre-registration pharmacist at the Royal Bournemouth General Hospital, where he had originally developed his interest in pharmacy following a period of work experience a number of years before. He then worked as a junior pharmacist at Southampton General Hospital where he went on to complete a clinical pharmacy diploma. An interest in Technical Services resulted in a move to the University Hospital of Wales, Cardiff, in November 2000. In 2004 he graduated from the University of Leeds with merit in Pharmaceutical Technology and Quality Assurance MSc. He is currently appointed as a senior pharmacist at Southampton General Hospital, specialising in clinical nutrition. Peter became a qualified Supplementary Prescriber in 2004 from King's College London and plays an active prescribing role on a daily basis within the adult Nutrition Team at Southampton. He also teaches and gives presentations on nutrition support and aspects of Technical Services. He has recently become the UK South West (East) regional British Association for Parenteral and Enteral Nutrition (BAPEN) representative as well as a member of the UK research and development subgroup of the Pharmaceutical Aseptic Services Committee.

Mike Stroud graduated in 1976 with a First-Class BSc in Human Biology from University College London, followed by qualifying in medicine at St George's Hospital London in 1979. Through the 1980s he interspersed working as junior hospital doctor with various polar expeditions before moving into full-time research on human performance physiology and becoming the Chief Scientist at the Government Centre for Human Sciences in 1993. In 1995, he returned to mainline medicine to work on clinical nutrition, initially as a Research Fellow in Southampton but later as Senior Lecturer in Medicine and Nutrition and a Consultant Gastroenterologist. He gained his MRCP in 1984 and was made a Fellow of the Royal Colleges of Physicians in both London and

Edinburgh in 1994. In 1996 he was awarded an MD for research work on the interactions between body weight, nutritional intake and exercise. He is a member of BAPEN Council and sits on both the Nutrition Committee and the Sports and Exercise Committee of the Royal Colleges of Physicians in London. He is also a member of the Small Bowel and Nutrition Committee of the British Society of Gastroenterology. Between 2003 and 2006, he was the chair of the National Institute for Health and Clinical Excellence (NICE) Guidelines development group on Nutrition Support. His main clinical and research interests are in intestinal failure, inflammatory bowel disease, malnourishment and nutrition support.

Abbreviations

AA   amino acid
ACE   angiotensin-converting enzyme
ALP   alkaline phosphatase
ALT   alanine transferase
AST   aspartate transferase
BAPEN   British Association for Parenteral and Enteral Nutrition
BMI   body mass index
BMR   basal metabolic rate
BNF   *British National Formulary*
BP   *British Pharmacopoeia*
CRP   C-reactive protein
CRS   catheter-related sepsis
CT   computerised tomography
CVC   central venous catheter
DEXA   dual-spectrum X-ray densitometry
ESR   erythrocyte sedimentation rate
ETF   enteral tube feeding
EVA   ethylene vinyl acetate
HEPA   high-efficiency particulate air
INR   international normalised ratio
IVN   intravenous nutrition
JVP   jugular venous pressure
LCT   long-chain triglyceride
MA   Marketing Authorisation
MCA   Medicines Control Agency
MCT   medium-chain triglyceride
MHRA   Medicines and Healthcare products Regulatory Agency
MUST   Malnutrition Universal Screening Tool
NICE   National Institute for Health and Clinical Excellence
NST   nutrition support team
PEG   percutaneous endoscopic gastrostomy
PEGJ   percutaneous endoscopic gastrostomy-jejunal

PICC	peripherally inserted central catheter
PL	Product Licence
PN	parenteral nutrition
PVC	polyvinyl chloride
PVT	peripheral vein thrombophlebitis
RCT	randomised controlled trial
RIG	radiologically inserted gastrostomy
RMR	resting metabolic rate
RNI	recommended nutrient intake
RQ	respiratory quotient
SALT	speech and language therapist
SBS	short-bowel syndrome
SCFA	short-chain fatty acid
SIADH	syndrome of inappropriate antidiuretic hormone
WBC	white blood cell count

1

The importance of nutrition support

Why worry about nutrition?

The importance of good nutrition in maintaining health and preventing disease is well recognised. Nevertheless, few people realize that malnutrition or the risk of becoming malnourished is a common threat to patients in UK clinical practice. In most cases, the cause of patient malnourishment is an illness-related change in the intake, metabolism, excretion or demand for nutrients. In some, however, there are also longer-standing background issues such as poverty and social isolation.

Any problems of malnutrition are often worsened on admission to hospital because investigation and routine pre- and postoperative management entail periods of 'nil by mouth' or restricted intake. Patients are also unable to feed themselves properly, miss meals when off the wards or do not like the hospital catering. Figure 1.1 shows the multiple factors that combine to pose a nutritional threat to patients with a wide variety of medical or surgical problems.

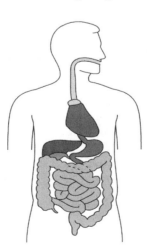

Altered nutrient processing
Increased/changed metabolic
    demands
Liver dysfunction

Impaired intake
Poor diet
Poor hospital catering
Poor appetite
Missed meals
Pain/nausea with food
Mucositis
Dysphagia
Depression/psychological
Unconscious

Excess losses
Vomiting
Nasogastric tube drainage
Diarrhoea
Surgical drains
Fistulae
Stomas

**Impaired digestion and
absorption**
    e.g. problems of
stomach, intestine,
pancreas and liver

Figure 1.1 Common causes of malnutrition in patients.

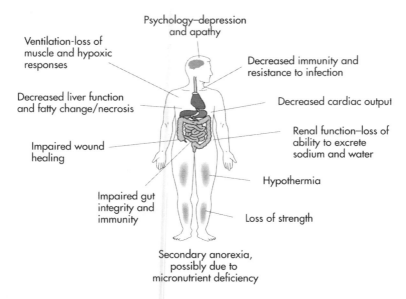

Psychology–depression and apathy

Ventilation-loss of muscle and hypoxic responses

Decreased immunity and resistance to infection

Decreased liver function and fatty change/necrosis

Decreased cardiac output

Impaired wound healing

Renal function–loss of ability to excrete sodium and water

Impaired gut integrity and immunity

Hypothermia

Loss of strength

Secondary anorexia, possibly due to micronutrient deficiency

Figure 1.2 The effects of malnutrition.

The effects of malnutrition

The ill effects of malnourishment include vulnerability to infection, poor wound healing, muscle weakness, depression and apathy as shown in Figure 1.2. All contribute to poor clinical outcomes. For example, studies in surgical patients show that the malnourished are 3–4 times more likely to have complications than their better-nourished counterparts undergoing the same operative procedure[1]. They also stay in hospital for around 5 days more, have higher mortality rates and incur around 50% greater costs[1].

Of course, not all of the poor clinical outcomes seen in malnourished patients can be ascribed to malnutrition *per se*. In many cases their underlying medical problems are more severe or have been present for longer. Nevertheless, studies of nutritional intervention illustrate that specifically treating malnutrition provides benefit. For example, simple measures to improve the oral intake of malnourished individuals have led to reductions in complication and mortality rates of 53% and 24% respectively[2]. Benefits derived from the more invasive and risky enteral tube and intravenous feeding techniques are less certain, mainly because randomised controlled trials cannot be conducted on ethical grounds if the invasive feeding method on trial is the only way to provide patients with the nutrients they need (see Chapter 3).

Who needs nutrition support?

In 2006, the UK National Institute for Health and Clinical Excellence (NICE) published guidelines on nutrition support[3]. These guidelines state that good health care should include the provision of adequate nutrition to meet all patients' needs. This can usually be achieved by good catering as long as care is taken to avoid missed meals and help with eating is provided when necessary. In some cases, however, good food alone cannot do the job. This is usually due to:

- Loss of appetite
- Diminished level of consciousness
- Inability to swallow safely
- Intestinal failure
- Excessive metabolic demands
- Excessive nutrient losses

In such cases nutrition support may be needed, with the overall aim that total intake (from normal food and drinks plus support) provides adequate energy, protein, electrolytes, micronutrients and fluid to meet the patients' needs. NICE recommends that support is considered for any patient who is underweight, losing weight or unable to eat for prolonged periods. The criteria used to define those who may need nutritional help are shown in Box 1.1.

If nutrition support is required, it should be given orally if possible, since this is usually effective, safe and cheap. If oral supplementation cannot be used safely or fails to meet a patient's needs, enteral tube feeding should be considered. However, in some patients this is also

---

Box 1.1 National Institute for Health and Clinical Excellence (NICE) recommendations on indications for nutrition support

Nutrition support should be considered in people who are malnourished or at risk of malnourishment, as defined by any of the following:

- A body mass index (BMI) < 18.5 kg/m^2
- Unintentional weight loss >10% in the last 3–6 months
- A BMI < 20 kg/m^2 and unintentional weight loss > 5% in the last 3–6 months
- People who have eaten little or nothing for > 5 days or are likely to eat little or nothing for the next 5 days or longer
- People with a poor absorptive capacity and/or high nutrient losses and/or increased nutritional needs from causes such as catabolism

unsafe, impossible or ineffective. It is in these groups that intravenous nutrition (IVN) will need to be considered.

Ethical issues in nutrition support

Artificial nutrition support is fraught with ethical and legal difficulties and all prescribers of IVN should be familiar with these. In general, providing adequate and appropriate fluid and nutrients is a basic duty to sick patients and while a patient can swallow and expresses a desire or willingness to drink or eat, fluid and nutrients should be given unless there is a medical contraindication. If the patient cannot safely consume or absorb adequate amounts orally, administration of nutrients and/or fluid via a tube or vein must be considered. Legally, however, this becomes a 'medical treatment' and hence can be withheld or withdrawn if providing or continuing such support is not in the patient's best interests. If, for example, an illness is regarded as being in the terminal phase and the plan is to provide only compassionate and palliative care, ethical considerations indicate that a tube/vein supply of nutrients or fluid need only be given to relieve symptoms and should not necessarily be used to prolong survival. In cases where benefits are in doubt, a planned time-limited trial of artificial feeding may be useful.

Whenever nutrition support is used, patients should give their consent and a competent patient's refusal is binding. If a patient lacks the competence to make a decision, the patient's doctor should seek to ascertain whether the patient expressed previous views about the type of treatment that he or she would wish to receive if the present state of incompetence occurred. If no such views can be identified, any decisions on tube or vein provision of food and/or fluids should involve consultation with the family and all members of the health care team. However, under current English law, relatives or a nominated proxy cannot make a decision on behalf of an adult patient and so cannot override the clinician's decision. Special considerations apply in relation to children and application to the court should be made regarding the legality of withdrawing artificial hydration and nutrition from a patient in a persistent vegetative state.

Under specified circumstances, it can be legal to enforce nutritional treatment for an unwilling patient with a mental disorder. This includes anorexia nervosa, in which it is considered that severe malnourishment *per se* can render patients incompetent of making rational decisions regarding their care.

A comprehensive overview of the legal position in the UK regarding the withholding or withdrawing of nutritional support can be found in the following references:

- Luttrell S. Withdrawing or withholding life prolonging treatment. *Br Med J* 1999; 318: 1709–1710.
- British Medical Association. *Withholding and Withdrawing Life-prolonging Medical Treatment: Guidelines for Decision Making*, 2nd edn. London: British Medical Journal Books, 2001.
- British Association for Parenteral and Enteral Nutrition. *Ethical and Legal Aspects of Clinical Hydration and Nutritional Support*. Maidenhead: British Association for Parenteral and Enteral Nutrition.

References

1. Lennard-Jones J. *A Positive Approach to Nutrition as Treatment*. London: British Association for Parenteral and Enteral Nutrition, 1992: 14.
2. Stratton R, Green C, Elia M. *Disease-Related Malnutrition: An Evidence Based Approach to Treatment*. Wallingford: CABI Publishing, 2003: 221–222.
3. NICE and the National Collaborating Centre For Acute Care. *Nutrition Support in Adults: Oral Nutrition Support, Enteral Tube Feeding and Parenteral Nutrition*. London: NICE and the National Collaborating Centre For Acute Care, 2006.

2

Oral and enteral tube support

Intravenous nutrition (IVN) should only be used in patients who cannot be supported by other methods. Prescribers of IVN must therefore understand the indications, benefits, limitations and risks of providing nutrition support by the oral route or enteral tube feeding.

Oral nutrition support

Oral nutrition support is usually the cheapest, safest and most physiological method of providing additional nutrition. At its simplest, the importance of eating to prevent problems and to aid recovery should be explained to patients with encouragement to eat all meals provided. Staff should also try to ensure that meals are not missed through investigations or procedures unless absolutely necessary. Needing to be nil by mouth for a gastroscopy is acceptable, but missing lunch because the patient was off the ward for a chest X-ray is not.

If spontaneous intake is felt to be inadequate, encouragement and help should be offered and records of daily food, nutritious drinks and other fluid intake should be commenced. If the problem then persists, dietetic advice should be sought. Some patients may benefit from special menus, snacks and increased choice, and dietitians are in an ideal position to explore these possibilities. Changing food consistency may also lead to improved intake in some patients with swallowing difficulties. Soft diets may help in oesophageal stricturing whereas thickened liquids may help patients with neurological dysphagia. Great care must be taken, however, to ensure that dysphagic patients who are allowed to continue with oral intake do not aspirate. Assessment by a speech and language therapist (SALT), with or without radiological assessment of swallowing, may be required.

Food fortification, using either high-energy foodstuffs (e.g. butter or cream) or commercially available energy and/or protein supplements, is commonly recommended to try to improve nutritional intake. We believe, however, that the use of this type of nutritional supplementation should be viewed with caution. Malnourished individuals are usually depleted in micronutrients, electrolytes and minerals *as well* as energy and protein, and food fortification may fail to address all of their needs. This could also put them at risk of a refeeding problem through shortage of a critical nutrient (see Chapter 9). We therefore recommend that oral supplementation beyond that provided from normal food should be with commercially produced, nutritionally complete protein, energy and micronutrient preparations, e.g. sip-feed drinks. Even then, some caution is needed. Although such commercial 'complete' supplements do contain sufficient quantities of vitamins and minerals to meet daily requirements, they only do so if patients are consuming enough of the supplement to meet their entire energy and protein needs. This is often not the case and patients are only using the supplement as additional intake above that from food. They may, therefore, still need additional multivitamin and trace element supplementation to ensure balanced and truly complete nutrient intake.

It is important that any oral nutritional supplements including, for example, sip-feed drinks and micronutrients, are prescribed on drug charts. This will not only ensure that they are actually given by nursing staff but also indicate clearly to both patients and staff that nutritional care is an integral part of medical treatment.

Types of oral supplement

Many types of oral nutrition supplement are available in a wide choice of flavours. Most are liquid sip-feeds but some come in other forms such as desserts. A full description of all types is beyond the remit of this book and advice from dietitians is often required. Nevertheless, the IVN prescriber should know the basics of what is available and understand the rationale behind different supplement use.

Most commercial oral supplements contain energy, protein, vitamins, trace elements and fluid, with some containing fibre. They are usually nutritionally complete if used alone to meet all of a patient's energy needs. Most contain 1.0 kcal/mL but higher-energy versions containing 1.5 kcal/mL are also available. Nitrogen content is usually equivalent to 4–6 g protein per 100 mL but they vary widely in energy-to-protein ratios, nitrogen form and content, and the type of fat that they contain. The following broad types are commonly used:

- *Polymeric complete*: polymeric feeds containing nitrogen as whole protein or long polypeptides are most commonly prescribed. The carbohydrate source is mostly partially hydrolysed starch and the fat is predominantly long-chain triglycerides (LCTs). These feeds tend to be either sweet, apparently milky drinks or savoury formulas. They are suitable for patients who have no significant digestive problems.

- *Polymeric fat-free*: some polymeric oral supplements contain no lipid. They are therefore less nutritionally complete but many patients prefer the fruit drink-type format, particularly if the drink is diluted with water to limit its sweetness.

- *Fibre-containing feeds*: many oral supplements are available in standard and fibre-enriched forms. The standard feeds contain little or no fibre and hence they lead to little or no short-chain fatty acid (SCFA) production in the colon. Fibre-enriched feeds theoretically increase SCFA availability in the colon, which may increase salt and water reabsorption and limit growth of pathogenic bacteria by lowering colonic pH. Their effectiveness, however, is probably marginal, especially if patients are on antibiotics which reduce colonic flora.

- *Predigested and elemental feeds*: these feeds contain nitrogen as either short peptides or, in the case of elemental diets, as free amino acids. Carbohydrate provides much of the energy content while the fat content varies in both quantity and the proportion provided as LCTs and medium-chain triglycerides (MCTs). The aim of 'predigested' feeds is to improve nutrient absorption but their effectiveness is usually limited to maldigestive problems (e.g. pancreatic disease) rather than malabsorptive states. Indeed, they should generally be avoided in patients with a short gut or patients with small-bowel fistulae since their high osmolality can cause excess movement of water into the gut and hence increased diarrhoeal losses.

- *Specialised disease-specific and pharmaconutrient feeds*: some very specialised disease-specific and pharmaconutrient supplements are available but the indications for their use are complex and beyond the remit of this book. Sodium-supplemented sip-feeds are not available commercially but can be very useful in the management of patients with high-output stomas who tend to become salt-depleted. Indeed, the use of such sodium supplementation can avoid the need for IVN in some patients and hence their use must be understood by IVN prescribers (see Chapter 10).

Table 2.1 Common indications for enteral tube feeding

Indication for feeding	Examples
Unconscious patient	Head injury, ventilated patient, encephalopathy
Swallowing disorder	Post cerebrovascular accident, multiple sclerosis, motor neurone disease, Parkinson's disease
Physiological anorexia	Liver disease (particularly with ascites), cancer cachexia, especially in malnourished patient due to undergo surgery (since supplementary feeding helps reduce postoperative complications)
Upper gastrointestinal obstruction	Pharyngeal tumour, oesophageal tumour/stricture, pyloric stenosis
Partial intestinal failure	Postoperative ileus, inflammatory bowel disease, short-bowel syndrome
Increased nutritional requirements	Intensive-care patient, cystic fibrosis, renal disease
Psychological problems	Severe depression or anorexia nervosa

Enteral tube feeding (ETF)

Nutrition support using an enteral tube feed is usually needed for patients in whom oral intake is unsafe or impossible due to swallowing difficulties or diminished levels of consciousness. However, it may also be used for patients who *can* take food orally but are unable to meet their needs; for example, patients who have limited gut absorptive function can benefit from slow overnight tube feeding to add to their intake through meals and snacks alone.

Common indications for ETF are listed in Table 2.1.

Types of enteral feeding tubes

A variety of different tubes can be used to provide ETF. Choosing the best option depends on factors including anatomy, clinical condition and the proposed/expected period of feeding. Figure 2.1 shows the choices available as well as the techniques to check that the tube is correctly positioned. This is essential if complications are to be avoided (see below). It is important to appreciate that many patients may be resistant to the idea of ETF, especially if they have had a large-bore, stiff naso-gastric tube in the past. It is therefore important when possible to talk

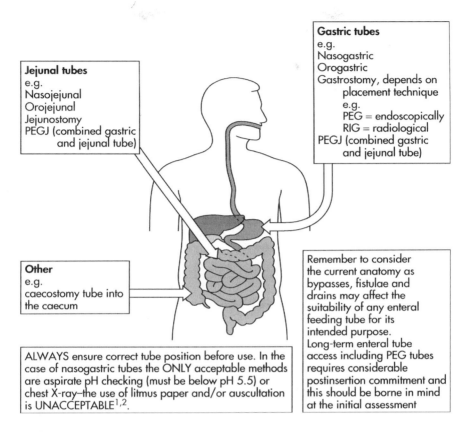

Jejunal tubes
e.g.
Nasojejunal
Orojejunal
Jejunostomy
PEGJ (combined gastric
        and jejunal tube)

Gastric tubes
e.g.
Nasogastric
Orogastric
Gastrostomy, depends on
        placement technique
        e.g.
        PEG = endoscopically
        RIG = radiological
PEGJ (combined gastric
        and jejunal tube)

Other
e.g.
caecostomy tube into
the caecum

Remember to consider
the current anatomy as
bypasses, fistulae and
drains may affect the
suitability of any enteral
feeding tube for its
intended purpose.
Long-term enteral tube
access including PEG tubes
requires considerable
postinsertion commitment and
this should be borne in mind
at the initial assessment

ALWAYS ensure correct tube position before use. In the
case of nasogastric tubes the ONLY acceptable methods
are aspirate pH checking (must be below pH 5.5) or
chest X-ray–the use of litmus paper and/or auscultation
is UNACCEPTABLE[1,2].

Figure 2.1 Enteral tube options.

through the type of tube proposed, its placement and plans for its subsequent use.

Nasogastric and orogastric tubes

Nasogastric or orogastric tubes are usually used in patients for short-term ETF (e.g. less than 4 weeks' duration). Feeding by this route allows the stomach to act as a reservoir to hold and release the feed at a steady rate, which minimises discomfort associated with feeding. However, delayed gastric emptying is common in patients with more severe illness and so nasogastric feeding is often poorly tolerated. Risks of aspiration are also high but can be reduced by feeding patients sat up at an angle of 30–45° and by keeping them propped up for at least 30 minutes after feeding. All modern nasogastric feeding tubes are soft and fine-bore (6–10 French gauge), which makes them relatively comfortable.

Nasojejunal tubes

Nasojejunal tubes are passed via the nose into the jejunum, lying beyond both the oesophagogastric and pyloric sphincters. This may reduce the risk of aspiration. Since the food bypasses the gastric acid barrier, feed sterility becomes very important and the loss of the gastric reservoir also means that delivery rates must be slow. Jejunal feeding is often used when there are known problems of gastro-oesophageal reflux or delayed gastric emptying, especially in unconscious patients who have to be nursed flat. The technique is also used in upper gastrointestinal surgical patients when the tube is inserted at the time of operation and left across oesophageal, gastric or duodenal anastamoses. Feed is then delivered distal to the vulnerable areas of surgical reconstruction. All nasojejunal tubes are also fine-bore (6–10 French gauge), with some having a shorter, second lumen for gastric aspiration.

Gastrostomy and jejunostomy tubes

Gastrostomy and jejunostomy tubes pass directly through the abdominal wall into the stomach or jejunum. Most are placed endoscopically (e.g. PEGs), although radiological placement is not uncommon and surgical placement is sometimes used. They tend to be utilised for patients requiring longer-term feeding or those in whom nasogastric passage is difficult to achieve. Aspiration, especially with gastrostomies, remains a risk and hence feed should still be given with the patient at an angle of 30–45° (see above) whenever possible.

Types of enteral feed

The choice of enteral tube feed is influenced by a patient's nutritional requirements, gastrointestinal function and the presence of other problems such as renal or liver impairment. As with oral sip supplements, most enteral feeds contain energy, protein, electrolytes, vitamins, trace elements and fluid, and most are nutritionally complete if they are used to fulfil a patient's entire energy needs. The majority contain 1.0 kcal/mL, but higher-energy versions containing 1.5 kcal/mL are also available. Nitrogen content is usually equivalent to 4 g protein per 100 mL but feeds vary widely in energy-to-protein ratios, osmolality, nitrogen form and content, and the type of fat they contain. Most come in liquid form and are ready to use straight from the container. As with oral supplements, polymeric, fibre-containing, predigested, elemental and pharmaconutrient versions are available (see above). Expert dietetic advice is often needed to ensure best-possible tolerance of ETF and hence to minimise the chances of treatment failure and the need for IVN.

Starting enteral tube feeding

If a dietitian is unavailable for advice, a standard feed should usually be used to start ETF, with the aim of gradual introduction of nutrition support. For patients at high risk of refeeding complications (see Chapter 8), starting rates as low as 5 or 10 mL/hour may be needed, in which case separate and generous electrolyte and vitamin replacement will usually be needed as well as additional fluids. In patients with no significant risk of refeeding problems, initial rates of around 20 kcal/kg per day may be used. Rates can then be increased to meet patients' full needs once it is established that the feeding is well tolerated.

Complications from enteral tube feeding

Everyone prescribing IVN should understand the problems and complications of ETF since many decisions on IVN use revolve around such limitations.

Common ETF problems are summarised in Table 2.2.

Tube insertion complications

Problems due to the insertion of fine-bore nasogastric or nasojejunal tubes are relatively uncommon but perforation of a pharyngeal or oesophageal pouch can occur and intracranial insertion has been reported. Perforation of the lower oesophagus, stomach or small bowel is sometimes seen, especially if the insertion guidewire is put back in and accidentally exits via a side port of the tube or punctures the wall of the tube where it is kinked. Stiffer polyvinyl and polypropylene tubes can cause perforation with no guidewire present.

Accidental bronchial placement of nasogastric and nasojejunal tubes is potentially very serious and is relatively common in patients with reduced levels of consciousness and/or impaired gag and swallowing reflexes. The presence of an endotracheal tube in a ventilated patient does not preclude bronchial insertion. In view of the risk, careful postplacement assessment of nasogastric tube position is needed using pH paper or chest X-ray checks (Figure 2.1). Clinical assessment of tube

Table 2.2 Complications of enteral tube feeding

Type	Complication
Tube insertion problems	Nasogastric and nasojejunal tubes – nasal damage, pharyngeal/oesophageal perforation, bronchial placement, variceal bleeding PEG/PEGJ insertions may cause bleeding, peritonitis and intestinal or colonic perforation
Postinsertion tube-related problems	Discomfort, erosions, fistulae and strictures Tube 'falls out' Bronchial administration of feed Tube blockage
Gastrointestinal intolerance	Gastro-oesophageal reflux Oesophagitis Aspiration Nausea, bloating and pain Diarrhoea
Metabolic disturbance	Refeeding syndrome Hyperglycaemia Fluid overload Electrolyte disturbance

PEG, percutaneous endoscopic gastrostomy; PEGJ, percutaneous endoscopic gastrostomy–jejunal.

position must be repeated whenever the tube is used to ensure that it has not become displaced. Nasogastric or nasojejunal tube insertion should probably be avoided for 3 days after acute variceal bleeding.

Problems related to the insertion of percutaneous gastrostomy and jejunostomy tubes include abdominal wall or intraperitoneal bleeding and bowel perforation. Free air is visible on X-ray in 38% of patients but significant surgical intervention is needed in fewer than 5%[3]. Very high postprocedure mortalities of up to 40% within 1 month have been reported[3], but this is mainly ascribable to the risks of the disease underlying the need for tube placement, e.g. dysphagic stroke. Nevertheless, it emphasises the need for all patients to be fully assessed before any decision is taken to place a gastrostomy or jejunostomy tube.

Postinsertion tube-related problems

Feeding tubes can cause local trauma and pressure-related problems. These include nasopharyngeal discomfort, sore mouth, thirst, swallowing difficulties and a hoarse voice. Mouthwashes, sucking ice cubes and using artificial saliva may help. Much less commonly, the tubes cause nasal erosion, abscess formation, sinusitis or otitis media. Avoiding large, stiff tubes helps and swapping the tube to the other nostril every 4–6 weeks also limits such problems. Local abrasion or gastro-oesophageal reflux may cause oesophagitis with potential stricturing if left untreated.

Displacement of nasally placed tubes is very common and about 25% of nasogastric tubes 'fall out' or are 'pulled out' by patients soon after insertion[3]. Tubes, especially if fine-bore, can also be displaced by coughing or vomiting. The biggest threat from displacement is that the feeding tube ends up in the oesophagus or bronchial tree, with consequent risk of aspiration. It is therefore essential to check the position of enteral tubes before each use (see above).

Postinsertion gastrostomy and jejunostomy tube complications include infection at the insertion site, peristomal leaks, accidental tube removal, tube fracture, gastrocolic fistula, peritonitis, septicaemia and necrotising fasciitis. PEGJ tubes can also fall back into the stomach or become disconnected, with the whole tube passing through the gut. Surgical jejunostomies should be left in for 3–5 weeks, even if feeding has stopped, so that a tract can become established and the pursestring suture holding the tube has dissolved.

Any enteral feeding tube can block, especially if not flushed before and after every feed or medication administered through it. Any drugs that are given through a tube should therefore be non-viscous elixirs or suspensions rather than syrups and should only be given after establishing compatibility. Hyperosmolar drugs, crushed tablets, potassium, iron supplements, sucralfate and preparations containing calcium, magnesium or phosphate are particularly likely to cause problems.

A tube can often be unblocked by flushing with warm water or, if this fails, by using an alkaline solution of pancreatic enzymes. Carbonated acidic drinks, pineapple juice and sodium bicarbonate solution should be avoided since they can cause tube degradation and worsen tube blockage[4,5]. Unlike nasogastric and nasojejunal tubes, gastrostomy tubes are sometimes occluded by gastric mucosal overgrowth ('buried bumper'). Loosening and rotating a gastrostomy tube at least once every week helps to prevent the problem. Further information on medicines and enteral tubes can be found in Chapter 5.

Gastrointestinal intolerance

Gastrointestinal intolerance of ETF is very common. Reflux of enteral feed into the oesophagus and potentially the lungs is frequent, especially in patients who need to be nursed flat on their back and those with impaired consciousness or poor gag reflexes. Problems occur in up to 30% of those with tracheostomies and 12.5% of neurological patients[3]. The reflux is probably caused by a combination of gravitational back-flow and impairment of gastro-oesophageal sphincter function due to pharyngeal stimulation from the tube and its position across the oesoph-agogastric junction. Aspiration can lead to life-threatening pneumonia and this may be 'silent' with no obvious vomiting or coughing. Acid suppression or sucralfate may help with symptoms of oesophagitis but does not prevent aspiration pneumonia.

Aspiration risks are increased if gastric residues accumulate and so feeding should be stopped or slowed if a 4-hour gastric aspirate is greater than 200 mL. Although continuous pump feeding reduces gastric pooling, it is often used overnight and hence any advantage over bolus or intermittent feeding may be offset. Overall, there is little difference in outcomes or complications using continuous, bolus or intermittent techniques[6]. Iso-osmotic feeds cause less delay in gastric emptying than high osmotic feeds and prokinetic drugs such as metoclopramide or erythromycin may be helpful. Postpyloric feeding makes aspiration less likely but does not eliminate the problem. PEG feeding only slightly reduces the risk of aspiration whereas jejunostomy feeding does reduce the relative risk.

Nausea and bloating occur in about 10–20% of ETF patients and ETF-related diarrhoea is seen in around 30% of those on medical and surgical wards and more than 60% of those on intensive care units[3]. The diarrhoea causes serious problems of nutrient, fluid and electrolyte loss and may also cause infected pressure sores and general distress. Causes of ETF diarrhoea are multiple and need to be thought through carefully before deciding whether a patient referred because of ETF diarrhoea really needs to start IVN. The causes include:

- *Feed delivery site and rate*: excessive feeding rates may cause gastrointestinal discomfort and diarrhoea, especially in the presence of poor gastric or small-bowel motility. Trying continuous rather than bolus feeding or vice versa may be helpful but there is no evidence that starter regimens with diluted or hypotonic diets are of value and these approaches can unnecessarily delay the provision of adequate nutrition.
- *Feed type*: although fibre-enriched feeds can normalise gastro-intestinal transit times, they rarely help with ETF-induced diarrhoea. Partially digested or elemental feeds can be useful in

patients with poor pancreatic digestive function but these should be avoided in patients with short-bowel problems due to their high osmolality. Increasing the sodium content of enteral feeds and low-fat feeds (or MCT fat feeds) may be helpful in such patients (see Chapter 10).

- *Drugs and ETF diarrhoea*: always check drug charts carefully when diarrhoea occurs with ETF and stop those which may be responsible whenever possible (see Chapter 5).
- *Infective causes*: enteral feed provides an ideal culture medium and, if contaminated, bacteria rapidly multiply. Stool samples must be checked whenever ETF patients develop diarrhoea.
- *Lactase deficiency*: primary lactase deficiency is common in many parts of the world and secondary deficiency can occur whenever there is gut damage from inflammation or infection. However, most commercial enteral feeds are lactose-free.
- *Hypoalbuminaemia*: there is debate over whether low albumin causes ETF diarrhoea through intestinal oedema. However, rather than a direct effect, it seems more likely that both low albumin and gut dysfunction reflect generalised membrane leakiness and fluid overload. Measures should therefore be taken to correct generalised oedema if possible and this should improve gastrointestinal function and hence limit the need for IVN.

If diarrhoea remains a problem after attention to all the above causes, high-dose loperamide can be tried and, if this fails, codeine phosphate. Feed rates can be reduced for a trial period but temporary IVN may be required. Constipation, with or without overflow, may also occur with ETF.

Metabolic complications of enteral tube feeding

Artificial feeding of patients by any method can cause metabolic problems, including deficiencies or excess of fluid, electrolytes, vitamins and trace elements. When commencing feeds in patients who have recently starved, there is a particular danger of inducing the refeeding syndrome (see Chapter 8). Overhydration also occurs frequently, particularly if patients are also receiving IVN or fluids.

Hyponatraemia is common when ETF is used in sicker patients. It is often accompanied by the development of oedema and is frequently related to the adverse effects of malnourishment and illness combined with excessive intravenous fluids such as 5% w/v glucose. Most patients have an excess of both body water and total body sodium and so treatment usually entails fluid restriction rather than increased sodium provision. Generous delivery of potassium to encourage cell membrane sodium exchange may also be helpful. Hypernatraemia due to excess water loss from transient diabetes insipidus may occur in neurosurgical or head-injury patients.

Between 10 and 30% of ETF patients are hyperglycaemic[3] and some may need oral antidiabetic agents or insulin. Rebound hypo-glycaemia is also seen if feeding is stopped abruptly, especially if patients are on antidiabetic therapy (see Chapter 10).

Conclusion

Oral supplementation and ETF are valuable means of providing nutrition support but they are not always effective and in some patients they cannot be used or cause complications. It is under those circum-stances that the use of IVN must be considered.

References

1.   Medicines and Healthcare products Regulatory Agency. *Medical Device Alert: Enteral Feeding Tubes (Nasogastric)*. London: MDA/2004/026; 14 June 2004.
2.   National Patient Safety Agency. *How to Confirm the Correct Position of Nasogastric Feeding Tubes in Infants, Children and Adults (interim advice)*. London: National Patient Safety Agency, February 2005.
3.   Stroud M, Duncan H, Nightingale J. Guidelines for enteral feeding in adult hospital inpatients. *Gut* 2003; 52 (suppl. VII): vii1–vii12.
4.   Smyth J, ed. *The NEWT Guidelines for Administration of Medication to Patients with Enteral Feeding Tubes or Swallowing Difficulties*. Wrexham: North East Wales NHS Trust, 2006: 10.
5.   Fair R, Proctor B. *Administering Medicines through Enteral Feeding Tubes*, 2nd edn. Belfast: The Royal Hospitals; 2004: 14.
6.   NICE and the National Collaborating Centre For Accute Care. *Nutrition Support in Adults: Oral Nutrition Support, Enteral Tube Feeding and Parenteral Nutrition*. London: NICE and the National Collaborating Centre For Acute Care, 2006.

3

Intravenous support

Who needs intravenous nutrition?

Intravenous nutrition (IVN) is needed if patients cannot meet their needs safely through oral and/or enteral tube feeding. The most common indication is intestinal failure in which the capacity of the gastro-intestinal tract to ingest and absorb food and/or fluid is inadequate to meet the body's needs. Intestinal failure can be acute or chronic, complete or partial, and reversible or irreversible.

Problems requiring IVN support are many and varied and examples of some of the more common indications are shown in Table 3.1. The table also includes examples of conditions which may necessitate nutrition support but in which other methods can generally be used.

IVN is sometimes needed in patients who probably do have adequate gastrointestinal absorptive function but in whom oral/enteral intake is unsafe and/or access for enteral tube feeding (ETF) cannot be achieved or maintained. In such cases, measures to try to gain stable tube access to the gut at a level compatible with safe feeding should be explored. For example, problems of patients pulling out enteral feeding tubes can usually be solved with adequate taping, repeated tube placements or by moving to feeding via a gastrostomy or jejunostomy. Occasionally, persistent diarrhoea caused by ETF does result in a requirement for IVN but all solvable causes of the problem should be excluded first (see Chapter 2). Nevertheless, if a patient has a relatively urgent need for nutrition support and successful ETF cannot be guaranteed swiftly, it is reasonable to start IVN while efforts to instigate or improve the success of enteral feeding are investigated.

Hypoalbuminaemia is not a marker of malnutrition and in itself is never an indication for IVN. It has been shown that IVN does not improve serum albumin over 10 days[1] and the failure of serum albumin to rise during a period of nutritional support should not be considered to reflect inadequacy of the nutrition provided[2].

Table 3.1 Potential support options for patients with nutritional problems

Nature of problem	Examples of problems	Potential nutritional management
Poor oral intake	Anorexia of disease	Problem can usually be overcome by using oral supplements or ETF: IVN is very rarely needed
	'Routine' nil by mouth after surgery	IVN may be indicated if restriction is likely to be prolonged and/or patient is already malnourished. You need to know: • How long oral restriction is envisaged • Whether and when ETF may be possible and whether it is likely to be safe and effective in the context of that patient's operation and the presence or absence of postoperative ileus
	Anorexia nervosa	Problem can usually be overcome using oral supplements or ETF, with great caution to avoid refeeding risks (see Chapter 8). IVN is only rarely indicated, if patient is at critical risk and refuses all other means of help
Swallowing difficulties – local or mechanical	Mucositis from chemotherapy/total body irradiation	This is a frequent indication for IVN, especially in patients receiving high-dose chemotherapy for haematological malignancy. Pain can preclude significant oral intake and prevent effective ETF because of tube intolerance or malabsorption/diarrhoea (from mucosal damage elsewhere in gastrointestinal tract)
	Oropharyngeal tumour with and without surgery, radiotherapy	ETF is usually possible, although IVN may be required until enteral tube is placed. Obstruction may prevent nasogastric tube placement and a gastrostomy feeding tube (often placed before surgery or irradiation) is very useful
	Pharyngeal pouch	A large pouch can cause dysphagia and make enteral tube access difficult. IVN may be needed as a temporary measure until enteral access is achieved

Table 3.1 Continued

Nature of problem	Examples of problems	Potential nutritional management
Swallowing difficulties – neurological	Stroke and bulbar or pseudobulbar palsy from motor neurone disease or multiple sclerosis	Dietary modification (often thickened fluids) or ETF can usually meet patients' needs but aspiration may be problematic. IVN may be needed while waiting for satisfactory enteral tube access. SALT assessment is needed
	Unconscious patient	ETF is usually feasible, although delayed gastric emptying may pose problems (especially in head injury or other causes of raised intracranial pressure). Motility agents or jejunal feeding can usually overcome problems but IVN may be needed until postpyloric access is established
Oesophageal problems	Benign stricture Malignant stricture Motility disorder	Dietary modification using puréed foods or liquid supplements may be effective but there is a risk of aspiration. ETF is usually possible but direct gastrostomy access, achieved either endoscopically or radiologically, may be needed. IVN is then used while waiting for either enteral tube access or treatment of obstruction by dilatation, stenting or surgery. SALT assessment may be needed
Stomach	Benign pyloric obstruction Malignant obstruction Gastric resection	IVN is often required while waiting for enteral tube access or treatment by dilatation, stenting or surgery. A postpyloric enteral tube placed endoscopically, radiologically or surgically may be needed. Patients who have a surgical bypass procedure or attempted curative gastric resections often require instigation or continuation of IVN postoperatively for prolonged ileus, especially if obstruction was due to malignancy
	Delayed gastric emptying	May lead to IVN requirement in postabdominal surgery patients, neurological patients and intensive-care patients with multiorgan failure. Postpyloric ETF is often tolerated but jejunal access can be difficult to achieve
Liver disease	Cirrhosis from any cause Acute liver inflammation or failure	Patients with liver disease are often malnourished and eat poorly but the use of oral supplements or ETF is usually adequate. IVN is occasionally needed when oral intake is negligible and ETF access is problematic or the enteral feed is poorly tolerated due to sepsis or ileus

(cont.)

Table 3.1 Continued

Nature of problem	Examples of problems	Potential nutritional management
Hepatobiliary and pancreatic surgery	Liver resection Pancreatic resection Cholecystectomy with complications	Hepatobiliary and pancreatic surgery often leads to protracted postoperative ileus, especially in patients with significant overall liver dysfunction who are prone to salt and water retention. Upper gastrointestinal anastomoses are also relatively vulnerable and many patients with liver and pancreatic problems are already malnourished prior to surgery. Maintaining adequate nutritional intake is therefore important, particularly following major liver resection when nutrient needs for regeneration are exceptionally high ETF is usually feasible especially if a nasojejunal tube is placed beyond both pylorus and vulnerable anastomoses before or during surgery. IVN may still be required, however, if there is persistent complete ileus or complications such as anastomotic leakage or fistulation. Postpancreatectomy patients may become diabetic
Pancreatic disease	Acute pancreatitis	IVN was traditionally used in all patients with pancreatitis in order to avoid oral or enteral intake which were thought to stimulate greater destructive release of pancreatic enzymes. Recently, however, it has been shown that ETF is safe and possibly better than IVN and hence intravenous feeding should only be used if there is a specific reason, such as severe ileus[3,4] or fistulation. Postpyloric feeding may be needed if there is delayed gastric emptying. Maldigestion may limit the absorption of standard enteral feeds and patients may also become diabetic
Small intestinal disease	Small-bowel strictures – malignant and benign Crohn's disease Chronic pseudo-obstruction Radiation enteropathy	Oral supplements and/or ETF can usually be used, although IVN may be needed if obstruction is severe or limited absorptive capacity leads to excessive gastrointestinal losses with oral/enteral nutrition. Extensive Crohn's (especially with multiple resections) and postradiation changes are common causes of chronic intestinal failure and the need for long-term home IVN

Table 3.1 Continued

Nature of problem	Examples of problems	Potential nutritional management
Post small intestinal surgery	Persistent ileus Extensive gut resection and short-bowel syndrome (see Chapter 10) Surgical complications such as anastomotic leak, fistulation or adhesions	IVN is often needed in such patients, especially if the patient is already significantly malnourished and so waiting for postoperative recovery of intestinal function is concerning. Extensive or multiple gut resections leading to short-bowel syndrome are common indications for long-term IVN support, especially after superior mesenteric artery infarct or multiple operations for Crohn's disease. Nearly all patients who have just become short-bowel patients need IVN for a period while they recover from surgery and the effectiveness of limited hypotonic fluid intake coupled with high-sodium drinks is evaluated (see Chapter 10). Abdominal surgery in the context of previous abdominal radiotherapy for any indication is particularly likely to result in prolonged postoperative ileus
Colonic disease	Ulcerative colitis Crohn's colitis Infective colitis	IVN is rarely required but in protracted illness, especially if surgery is likely to be needed, nutrition support is indicated and oral or enteral intake may worsen abdominal pain and diarrhoea. IVN may therefore be required and complete gut rest is also advocated in some cases of severe Crohn's disease, especially if there is fistulation
Colonic surgery	Colonic resection	Most colonic surgery patients requiring nutrition support can have oral or enteral feeding since severe persistent ileus is less common than with upper gastrointestinal surgery and lower gastrointestinal anastomoses are relatively strong. Nevertheless, IVN is sometimes needed, especially if there has been any peritoneal contamination or excessive postoperative salt and water have led to gut dysfunction

ETF, enteral tube feeding; IVN, intravenous nutrition; SALT, speech and language therapist.

Nutrition support in the surgical patient

Since the primary indication for IVN is intestinal failure, it is inevitably used most frequently in general surgical patients. In our experience, more than 60% of referrals for IVN are in this group, with persistent postoperative ileus being the commonest reason for IVN need. Persistent ileus is particularly likely to occur in patients who have become oedematous due to excessive salt and water administration. Some surgical patients have also lost so much weight preoperatively that they already qualify for nutrition support and IVN may be the only route available. Other postoperative complications, such as anastomotic leaks and the development of early adhesions, are also relatively common indications for IVN. It is therefore essential that all IVN prescribers understand the indications for IVN in pre-, peri- and postoperative situations.

Preoperative nutrition

Although studies show that active supplementary preoperative nutrition support is not helpful in all surgical patients, there is evidence of clear benefit in severely malnourished individuals[5]. Although benefits of preoperative feeding may be offset by disadvantages in delaying surgery, even short periods of 24–72 hours of improved nutrient intake probably correct some intracellular deficits of energy, potassium and micro-nutrients and hence grant improvements in resistance to infection, wound healing and muscle strength. Simple oral nutritional supplementation can be undertaken at home in malnourished, elective surgical patients who are awaiting admission, as long as they can swallow safely and do not have intestinal failure. Inpatient nutrition support using ETF or IVN can then be reserved for those with partial or complete intestinal failure. Feeding into the gut should be used whenever possible, although this may be restricted by problems such as obstruction or the practical requirements of preoperative gut preparation.

We therefore recommend that:

- Preoperative ETF is considered for malnourished patients (body mass index (BMI) < 18.5, weight loss > 10%) with inadequate or unsafe oral intake, who have a functional, accessible gastro-intestinal tract.
- Preoperative IVN is considered for malnourished patients (BMI < 18.5, weight loss > 10%) with an inadequate or unsafe oral intake and a non-functional or inaccessible gastrointestinal tract.

Patients should receive at least 3 days of preoperative nutrition support whenever possible and 7–10 days should be used in very malnourished patients (BMI < 16 and/or weight loss > 15%).

Perioperative nutrition

Major surgery invariably leads to acute physiological stress. Initially there may be suppression of metabolism which may last for 24 hours or more, followed by a catabolic response for several days. These processes are incompletely understood but nutrient utilisation during the initial phase is probably impaired, while during the catabolic phase the nutrient requirements for acute-phase proteins and mounting an immune response are probably different from those usually needed. Furthermore, many patients become very insulin-resistant, which further impairs nutrient utilisation (see Chapter 10). We therefore recommend very cautious approaches to feeding during and immediately after surgery. In particular, we suggest that:

- Feeding, even using IVN, should be stopped immediately prior to any major operation with a check of blood glucose in case of rebound hypoglycaemia.
- Recommencement of nutritional intake by any route should be delayed for 24 hours following a major operation, again checking blood glucose.

Early postoperative nutrition

Commencing or recommencing nutrition support at 24–48 hours post-surgery is recommended for all severely malnourished patients (BMI < 16 and/or > 15% weight loss) as well as for patients in whom a prolonged period of postoperative nutritional restriction seems inevitable. In all cases, nutrition should be commenced at a maximum of around 50% of estimated requirements for the first 24 hours (see Chapter 7), with even slower starting regimens in the severely malnourished who need careful clinical and biochemical monitoring to limit problems of refeeding syndrome (see Chapters 8 and 9) or stress-induced insulin resistance and hyperglycaemia (see Chapter 10).

There is considerable debate regarding the benefits of early, elective ETF after surgery. The National Institute for Health and Clinical Excellence (NICE) concluded, however, that there is no good evidence for this practice and hence that early postoperative ETF should only be

Table 3.2 Nutrition before and after major surgery

Day	Acceptable nutritional status	Malnourished (BMI < 18.5; weight loss > 10%; or BMI < 20 and weight loss > 5%)	Severely malnourished (BMI < 16; weight loss > 15%, or BMI < 18.5 and weight loss > 10%)
Preoperative	Avoid oral restriction when possible	Avoid oral restriction when possible. Consider oral nutrition support	Avoid oral restriction when possible. Consider pre-operative ETF or IVN, ideally for 7–10 days but at least 3 days if longer is impractical. Beware refeeding problems
Operation day + day 1 postoperative	Do not feed	Do not feed	Do not feed
Day 2 postoperative	Introduce oral intake at up to 50% of requirements if ready	Introduce oral intake at up to 50% of requirements if ready	Aim to meet 25–50% of requirements using oral intake if ready or ETF/IVN. Beware refeeding problems
Day 3 postoperative	Continue intake or introduce oral intake at up to 50% of requirements if ready	Aim to meet 50% of requirements using oral intake if possible. Consider ETF/IVN if oral intake inadequate	Increase nutrient intake slowly
Day 4 postoperative	Continue or introduce oral intake at up to 50% of requirements if ready	Slowly increase intake	Meet at least 50% of full requirements by oral, ETF or IVN routes alone or in combination
Day 5 postoperative	Meet 50% of requirements through oral intake if ready. Consider ETF or IVN if oral intake is inadequate	Meet full requirements	Increase intake
Day 6 postoperative	Increase intake	Meet full requirements	Meet full requirements
Day 7 postoperative	Meet full requirements	Meet full requirements	Meet full requirements

BMI, body mass index; ETF, enteral tube feeding; IVN, intravenous nutrition.

used in those who meet the general criteria for the instigation of nutrition support (i.e. they are malnourished or at risk of malnourishment) unless in the context of clinical trial to try to explore the value of this approach more thoroughly[7].

There is also considerable debate as to the advantages of ETF compared to IVN in patients who need nutrition support postoperatively. It is now recognised that many of the traditional limitations to postoperative ETF given nasogastrically can be avoided if feeding is given via nasojejunal tubes or intraoperatively placed jejunal tubes. These then allow feed to be administered directly into the small intestine, which is often working within 24 hours of an operation even if postoperative ileus is still affecting gastric and colonic function (which may take several days to recover). Absent bowel sounds are not a contraindication to jejunal feeding but, although postoperative ETF has several advantages over IVN, some surgeons have concerns about its safety. Anastomoses involving stomach, small bowel, biliary tree or pancreas are relatively vulnerable for the first few days and, although the possible superiority of ETF over IVN is often ascribed to maintained gut integrity, the evidence that IVN causes either villous atrophy or increased bacterial translocation is poor. The relative benefit of ETF under these circumstances may therefore relate to problems of early overfeeding when IVN is used, rather than a real advantage of ETF (see Chapter 7). As a result, we suggest that if postoperative nutrition support is needed, it is provided by the oral or enteral route whenever possible but that IVN is used if those routes are unsafe or unlikely to be effective. A summary of our resulting approach to perioperative nutrition is shown in Table 3.2.

Long-term IVN

Some patients with chronic intestinal failure require long-term intravenous feeding and may undertake this at home. Box 3.1 shows examples of the types of problem that lead to this need.

Any request to commence a patient on home IVN needs careful consideration as it is a significant undertaking and may not be appropriate or practical. Assessment should be undertaken within an experienced centre with expert staff since patients need very specific training and, on top of the usual risks of IVN (see Chapter 12), there are many issues related to service organisation and funding. Arranging home IVN usually takes skilled staff several weeks. Full details on home IVN are beyond the remit of this book, although some aspects are considered

---

Box 3.1 Examples of some potential indications for home intravenous nutrition

---

Short-bowel syndrome due to mesenteric artery infarct or Crohn's disease with multiple resections (see Chapter 10)

Chronic gut damage from previous radiation therapy

Chronic gut dysmotility

Palliative use in patients with gastrointestinal obstruction due to cancer (unusual in the UK)

---

elsewhere in the text. More information on chronic intestinal failure and the need for home IVN can be found in:

- Messing B, Hebuterne X, Nightingale J. Home enteral and parenteral nutrition for adults. In: Nightingale J, ed. *Intestinal Failure*. London: Greenwich Medical Media, 2001: 407–430.
- Leach Z. Organising home parenteral nutrition. *Br J Home Healthcare* 2005; 1: 7–9.

Venous access

All IVN needs to be administered through a dedicated intravenous feeding line using volumetric pumps with in-line air alarms. Patients therefore need suitable intravenous access and the routes used include:

- Centrally inserted venous catheters (CVCs)
- Peripherally inserted central venous catheters (PICCs)
- Specialised, fine-bore peripheral catheters which extend into larger more central veins (midlines)
- Truly peripheral catheters (i.e. cannulas) moved frequently to different veins in order to limit problems of peripheral vein thrombophlebitis
- Subcutaneous ports used for long-term IVN administration

Central venous catheters

The majority of patients supported by IVN are fed through a CVC. Selection criteria for this route of feeding include:

- The patient already has a suitable CVC with a port which can be used solely for feeding (for example, a postoperative patient with a CVC that was placed at the time of operation).

- The patient is likely to require IVN for a period of more than 2 weeks.
- Patients who have no suitable vein for peripheral feeding line placement.
- Patients requiring specialised feeds that cannot be given into smaller peripheral veins (for example, lipid-free or restricted-volume feeds that have high concentrations: see Chapter 7).

Any type of CVC can be used for IVN but one lumen must be dedicated to this purpose. This minimises the likelihood of infection (see Chapter 12). If IVN is likely to be continued for a prolonged period, aspects such as increased likelihood of infection, line comfort and likelihood of line dislodgement must be considered. We therefore suggest that if IVN is likely to be used for more than 2 weeks, it should ideally be given via a single lumen line into a subclavian vein, preferably run through a sub-cutaneous tunnel.

Many patients referred for IVN already have central venous access, usually in the form of a temporary internal jugular or subclavian line. Many of these have multiple lumens but there is considerable debate as to whether it is acceptable to utilise a free lumen in an existing line for dedicated IVN provision. Some experts suggest that a brand new clean catheter must be used whereas others permit the use of a lumen that has already been utilised, especially since line replacement carries some risks[6]. We recommend that, if a multiple-lumen central line is already in place, it should not be routinely changed before IVN is started unless there is a specific reason to do so. This is in line with NICE recommendations[7]. However, if an existing line may be infected, a new line will be required or IVN will need to be delayed until any infection is controlled (see Chapter 12).

Peripherally inserted central venous catheters

Peripherally inserted central catheters (PICCs) are usually placed in a large forearm vein but are long enough for the tip to lie in the superior vena cava. They are often used for prolonged chemotherapy or antibiotic administration but can also be used to administer IVN, offering the advantage that the catheter tip lies in a large central vein, but with fewer insertion risks than either the subclavian or internal jugular approaches. They therefore provide an alternative to a tunnelled, centrally sited catheter but probably increase the risks of venous thrombosis affecting the arm. They are not really suitable for home IVN since they affect the patient's dexterity. Their placement can also be difficult if the patient has poor peripheral veins or is particularly oedematous.

Specialised, fine-bore peripheral catheters which extend into larger more central veins (midlines)

Until recently it was thought that the risks of thrombophlebitis always limited the use of peripherally administered IVN. It is now recognised, however, that full intravenous feeding can be achieved in most patients by using lipid-containing feeds (with relatively low osmolality) given via narrow-gauge, non-irritant catheters (22 or 23 Fr polyurethane) which are placed in an antecubital vein but which are long enough to have their tip lying in the larger axillary vein (Plate 1). These catheters can be placed easily, generally last for more than a week and avoid most of the risks and costs of central-line placement. If phlebitis or infection occurs, the lines can often be replaced easily. They are not generally suitable, however, for patients likely to require IVN for more than 2 weeks and hence usual criteria for their placement include:

- No suitable pre-existing central access
- Patients must have reasonable antecubital veins
- A likely requirement for IVN of less than 2 weeks

Most of these midline feeding catheters are sited in the antecubital fossa using a Seldinger technique. They can be inserted on the ward but must be placed using a strict aseptic technique with adequate skin preparation, for example using 0.5% chlorhexidine in 70% methylated spirits. These catheters tend to last longer in the basilic vein compared to the cephalic vein.

Truly peripheral catheters

Sometimes it is useful to start IVN through a simple peripheral cannula while awaiting placement of a more suitable, longer-lasting line. In such cases a small, pink (20 Fr) or blue (22 Fr) peripheral cannula should be used for a maximum of 24 hours IVN administration[8] before changing to a new peripheral administration site or to one of the other access techniques described above. This practice is not advised in the routine management of patients unless specialised advice is available locally. Administration of lipid-free or low-volume IVN regimens through a peripheral cannula is not advised, although some pharmacological techniques may reduce the incidence of thrombophlebitis (see Chapter 12).

Some units do give IVN for longer periods through peripheral cannulae[9], putting arrangements in place to ensure that the administration site is changed every 24 hours, with peripheral veins used in rotation. However, although this has the advantage of being less invasive than central catheter placement, repeated cannulation is uncomfortable for the patient and running such a service requires considerable resources.

Tunnelled cuffed catheters and subcutaneous ports

If feeding is likely to be continued for more than 2 months or to be undertaken at home, IVN should be given via a cuffed, subcutaneously tunnelled subclavian catheter or a suitable subcutaneous port. Cuffed lines incorporate a rough Dacron-covered segment (the cuff) on the part of the line which ends up lying within the subcutaneous tunnel between the vein entry site and the skin exit site. Subcutaneous tissue grows into the cuff and hence limits the risk of the line being unintentionally pulled out. It may also reduce the chances of any infection tracking up the tunnel from the skin exit site and entering the circulation. However, the latter has little, if any, impact on episodes of catheter-related sepsis, since infection usually enters the system via the lumen after contamination during manipulation of the line hub.

Subcutaneous ports consist of a small, hollow stainless-steel chamber placed surgically beneath the skin, usually in the pocket of subcutaneous tissue just below the clavicle on the right or left chest wall. The port chamber is linked to a tunnelled central catheter which usually runs into a subclavian vein and has a specialised rubber diaphragm on the surface lying beneath the skin. This diaphragm can be repeatedly needled from the skin surface in order to gain central catheter access as required whilst, if the needle is removed, all external links from the central vein to the surface disappear. Local anaesthetic gel is often applied to the skin over the port diaphragm for about 30 minutes before a special, sterile, hollow needle is put through the skin and diaphragm to access the chamber and hence the central catheter. Vascuports have cosmetic benefits over more traditional intravenous access, allow patients to have a less restricted lifestyle than a tunnelled, cuffed line and reduce problems of line exit site infections. However, if they become infected it is almost impossible to sterilise them with antibiotics and they need surgical removal. They must only be accessed by fully trained patients or specially skilled staff using full aseptic technique.

Complications of intravenous nutrition

Complications of IVN include:

- Intravenous access-related trauma such as pneumothorax, arterial puncture, brachial nerve injury
- Air embolus
- Catheter-related infection and associated sepsis
- Thrombophlebitis of smaller veins
- Venous thrombosis of larger veins and the risk of pulmonary embolus
- Metabolic and biochemical disturbances

Details of these problems are given in Chapter 12: information on how to avoid such problems is contained in Chapters 6 and 11 in terms of patient assessment and prescribing and Chapter 13 in terms of clinical review, avoidance of infection and laboratory monitoring. Guidance on the treatment of IVN-related complications including occlusion, infection and thrombosis is given in Chapter 12.

Combined routes of nutrition support

The use of IVN does not preclude the concurrent use of oral intake or ETF and combined routes of nutrition support may be beneficial. For example, patients with mucositis are usually permitted to take things by mouth but their intake may be negligible due to pain. ETF or IVN is then required but, as the mucositis resolves, the patient can often slowly increase oral intake. In such cases the aim should be that the total level of nutrition consumed or provided is appropriate for the patient's needs (see Chapter 7). The practicalities of using more than one route of nutrient intake are considered in Chapter 16.

Does intravenous nutrition work?

It is self-evident that a severe decline in nutritional status will eventually affect a patient's clinical outcome and may even cause death. There is therefore no doubt that IVN is needed by patients who, for prolonged periods, cannot maintain adequate nutrient intakes by any other means. This is the group in which IVN is mostly used. Since it is unethical to withhold nutrition support in such cases (unless there is no hope of survival with a reasonable quality of life) there have been no randomised controlled trials (RCTs) to test the benefits of IVN in these circumstances. Instead, the only RCTs examining the potential benefits of IVN have been performed on patients at less extreme risk of malnutrition. They are thus studies on the elective use of IVN in patients who do not *really* need it. The results may therefore not apply to patients in whom the technique is usually used. A number of other problems also make interpretation of IVN trials difficult. These include:

- Trials have been undertaken in widely varying groups, with varied nutritional risks, in many different settings. The applicability of results across patient groups is therefore unclear.
- It is not usually feasible (or ethical) to have 'no nutrition' as a control arm in a trial.
- Patients in control groups of nutrition trials have often ended up on IVN if their problems have been prolonged.
- In many trials, the nutrition support in the treatment arms has been provided at levels which many experts now think of as potentially harmful in very sick or malnourished patients (see Chapter 7).

In the light of the above, it is not possible to draw firm, evidence-based conclusions about the effectiveness of IVN. Nevertheless, it is undoubtedly life-saving for patients who are at extreme nutritional risk.

References

1. Gogos C, Kalfarentzos F, Zoumbos N. Effect of different types of total parenteral nutrition on T-lymphocyte subpopulations and NK cells. *Am J Clin Nutr* 1990; 51: 119–122.
2. Fuhrman M, Charney P, Mueller C. Hepatic proteins and nutrition assessment. *J Am Diet Assoc* 2004: 104: 1258–1264.
3. Powell J, Murchison J, Fearon K *et al*. Randomized controlled trial of the effect of early enteral nutrition on markers of the inflammatory response in predicted severe acute pancreatitis. *Br J Surg* 2000; 87: 1375–1381.
4. Windsor A, Kanwar S, Barnes E *et al*. Compared with parenteral nutrition, enteral feeding attenuates the acute phase response and improves disease severity in acute pancreatitis. *Gut* 1998; 42: 431–435.
5. The Veterans Affairs Total Parenteral Nutrition Cooperative Study Group. Perioperative total parenteral nutrition in surgical patients. *N Engl J Med* 1991; 325: 525–532.
6. Gil R, Kruse J, Thill-Baharozian M, Carlson R. Triple- vs single-lumen central venous catheters. *Arch Intern Med* 1989; 149: 1139–1143.
7. NICE and the National Collaborating Centre For Acute Care. *Nutrition Support in Adults: Oral Nutrition Support, Enteral Tube Feeding and Parenteral Nutrition*. London: NICE and the National Collaborating Centre For Acute Care, 2006.

8.   Payne-James J, Khawaja H. First choice for total parenteral nutrition: the peripheral route. *J Parenteral Enteral Nutr* 1993; 17: 468–478.
9.   May J, Murchan P, MacFie J *et al*. Prospective study of the aetiology of infusion phlebitis and line failure during peripheral parenteral nutrition. *Br J Surg* 1996; 83: 1091–1094.

4

Clinical history and examination

Introduction

Careful assessment of all patients referred for intravenous nutrition (IVN) is essential in order to understand their nutritional requirements and how they might best be met. Your assessment must gather information on the patients' past and present nutrient intakes, whether their gastrointestinal tracts are accessible and working, and whether their metabolic requirements are unusual. You also need to know whether there are any problems with heart, lung, kidney, liver or pancreatic function, and whether any other issues might influence electrolyte, fluid and nutrient requirements. The presence of infection can also influence your decision on whether nutrition support is appropriate and the safest means of providing it.

A full clinical assessment of a patient referred for possible IVN comprises the following:

- Patient's details and reason for referral
- A nutritional/gastrointestinal-oriented clinical history from the referring team and notes
- A review of laboratory results
- A focused, clinical examination of the patient, including clarification of history and possibilities for suitable intravenous access
- A review of fluid balance and nutrient intake charts
- A review of all prescription charts (see Chapter 5)

Once you have this information, you can decide whether artificial nutrition support is necessary and whether it should be given orally, enterally or intravenously (see Chapters 2 and 3). You will also be able to determine the patient's likely needs in terms of energy, nitrogen, fluid, electrolytes, trace elements and vitamins (see Chapters 7–9).

NUTRITION TEAM REFERRAL

Date			Time	

Patient	
	Name
	Hospital number
	Date of birth
	Ward
	Consultant

Venous access

Referral by	
	Name
	Position
	Bleep
	Extension

Request for

Received by

Assessment

Review	
	Referral appropriate
	Enteral nutrition support
	Intravenous nutrition support
	No nutrition support
	Nutritional advice given to staff
	Nutritional advice given to patient

Additional notes

Figure 4.1 Nutrition team referral form.

Patient details and reason for referral

When taking an initial referral for nutrition support, always record patients' details, including name, age, identification number and location. Ask about the background to the case and enquire particularly about *why* they may need artificial nutrition. Try to ascertain whether they are most likely to need oral, enteral or IVN support so that the most appropriate member of the nutrition support team can review the patient. Respect the judgement of the referring team on this point but bear in mind that not all patients referred for IVN actually need it and many will be better served by a different method. Whatever the outcome of the referral, the reasons for your advice must be clearly stated and documented. If you advise against IVN, review the patient over the next few days to check whether your opinion proved to be correct.

A log is an excellent way of keeping track of referrals and subsequent outcomes and an example is shown in Figure 4.1. Data collection and review are discussed in more detail in Chapter 14.

Taking a clinical history

A history to evaluate the need for nutrition support differs from a standard medical history. The aim is to:

*   Discover whether patients' nutrient intake from food and any current nutrition support is likely to be meeting their needs
*   Understand their present and likely future capability to ingest, absorb and process nutrients
*   Establish whether there are other medical problems such as major organ dysfunction or the presence of infection that will influence your actions

You can usually obtain most of the information you need from the notes and/or members of the referring clinical team. Details and omissions can then be clarified with the patient.

History of nutrient intake and body weight change

As outlined in Chapter 1, decisions on providing any form of nutrition support are dependent on whether patients are underweight or losing weight and whether they have been or will be able to eat adequately. You therefore need to ask yourself the series of questions, detailed below.

What has happened to the patient's body weight?

Body weight accounting for height (body mass index: BMI) and percentage body weight change are good markers of net nutritional status. You must therefore determine what has happened to these parameters during the months leading up to the current problems. This can be surprisingly difficult. Case notes often say little or nothing about body weight and since many patients referred for IVN either have been or are acutely ill, they may not know or cannot tell you about any weight changes. It can also be difficult actually to weigh the patient. Ward scales are often missing or inaccurate and, even when weights are available, changes may reflect abnormal fluid status rather than changes in body tissue. Any recorded variation must therefore account for dehydration or overhydration, especially if frank oedema or ascites is present (see below). Often one is left with little more information than a broad idea from the patient or nursing staff that significant weight loss has occurred.

Have long-term issues affected the patient's nutrient intake?

Some patients have eaten poorly for prolonged periods before their current illness. This may be documented in the medical notes but usually you need to ask the patient. Examples of such long-term intake issues include patients who are vegetarian or gluten-intolerant and those who follow religious dietary restrictions. Chronic disease can also alter long-term intakes by causing general anorexia or symptoms that limit eating, such as the pain or nausea from strictures in patients with Crohn's disease. Living off fast foods or drinking too much alcohol also limits vitamin intake which can then inhibit healing and increase the risks of complications such as the refeeding syndrome or Wernicke-Korsakoff syndrome (see Chapters 8 and 9).

How much nutrition has the patient had recently?

Checking the adequacy of a patient's recent total nutrient intake from food, oral supplements and enteral tube feeding (ETF) is a fundamental determinant of whether they need IVN. Once again, however, although it is usually easy to establish that the intake has been zero or close to zero (for example, nothing since the day before surgery), it can be extremely difficult to determine how much intake has been achieved when the patient has been receiving *some* food, oral supplements or ETF. In such cases, try looking through the medical and nursing notes, asking for any feeding charts (see below) and quizzing both the patient and their nursing staff.

If ETF has or is already being used, you must determine whether it has caused complications or whether there have been any limitations to its use. These will also influence decisions on the need for IVN.

Has the patient already had any IVN?

It is not unusual to receive an IVN referral for a patient who has already received some intravenous feeding either in another hospital or elsewhere in your own, e.g. on the intensive care unit. You still need to consider, however, whether you would have prescribed IVN and whether it is still indicated. You must also determine exactly what the patient has received and for how long.

History of gastrointestinal function

Most patients needing IVN have intestinal failure or a gastrointestinal tract that cannot be accessed or safely used. Your history must therefore establish whether the patient can eat, drink, swallow, digest and absorb food and fluids effectively. You also need to know whether any gastrointestinal problems are acute or chronic, and whether time or any medical or surgical manoeuvre is likely to overcome them. Ask the following questions:

Have there been any long-standing problems of gastrointestinal function?

Some patients have had gastrointestinal problems that have limited their intake, digestion or absorption of food over prolonged periods and these may have started before the medical or surgical issues that led to this referral for nutrition support. Examples include long-standing Crohn's disease, previous gastrointestinal surgery, pancreatic dysfunction or untreated coeliac disease.

What has happened to gastrointestinal function during the period of recent illness or surgical intervention?

Your history must establish a broad picture of all that has happened to gastrointestinal function during the days or weeks of illness leading up to the IVN referral. This includes not only all recent history of problems with eating, swallowing, nausea, vomiting and abdominal pain but also any history of excess losses via diarrhoea, wounds, drains or high stomal outputs. Furthermore, you also need to identify all operative interventions and to know whether there are any current problems of oropharyngeal, oesophageal, gastric or intestinal function.

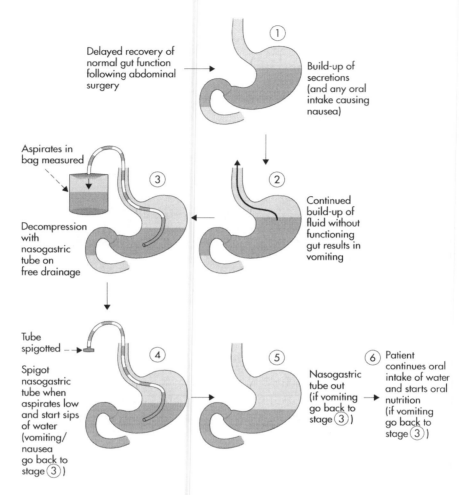

Delayed recovery of normal gut function following abdominal surgery → ① Build-up of secretions (and any oral intake causing nausea)

② Continued build-up of fluid without functioning gut results in vomiting

③ Aspirates in bag measured

Decompression with nasogastric tube on free drainage

④ Tube spigotted → Spigot nasogastric tube when aspirates low and start sips of water (vomiting/nausea go back to stage ③)

⑤ Nasogastric tube out (if vomiting go back to stage ③)

⑥ Patient continues oral intake of water and starts oral nutrition (if vomiting go back to stage ③)

Figure 4.2 Postoperative ileus.

A typical example of impaired gastrointestinal function is post-operative ileus and its delayed recovery is likely to account for the majority of your referrals for IVN (Figures 4.2 and 4.3).

Are the current gastrointestinal problems likely to resolve?

Once you know which parts of the gastrointestinal tract are not working, you can assess whether time or any therapeutic intervention is likely to improve them. The time since surgery and the presence of any postoperative complications are particularly critical in this evaluation. If the restriction on using the gut is simply to protect potentially

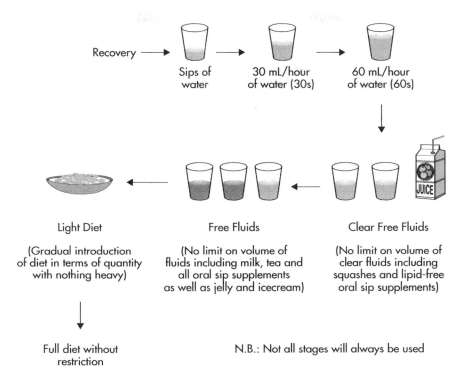

Recovery → Sips of water → 30 mL/hour of water (30s) → 60 mL/hour of water (60s)

Light Diet

(Gradual introduction of diet in terms of quantity with nothing heavy)

Free Fluids

(No limit on volume of fluids including milk, tea and all oral sip supplements as well as jelly and icecream)

Clear Free Fluids

(No limit on volume of clear fluids including squashes and lipid-free oral sip supplements)

Full diet without restriction

N.B.: Not all stages will always be used

Figure 4.3 Stages of return to full oral diet following surgery.

vulnerable anastamoses, the surgical team should be able to tell you when they envisage resumption of gastrointestinal use. Similarly, if any further surgery is planned, they may know the likely date, although you should bear in mind that any further intervention could precipitate a greater need for IVN rather than resolve the situation. Furthermore, having any surgery after a prolonged period of no nutrition is best avoided since healing of wounds and anastomoses may be compromised (see Chapter 3).

Any plans for the placement of an enteral feeding tube can also dictate whether IVN is required at the time of referral. In many cases, however, the likely time to resolution of gastrointestinal problems or attainment of enteral access is uncertain. This is particularly true with persistent postsurgical ileus, especially if it is related to complications such as an anastomotic leak or fluid overload. When there is such uncertainty, there is often little choice but to commence IVN in case the problems that prevent other means of feeding are slow to resolve. Importantly, however, if the need for IVN then proves to be short-lived, this should not be viewed as mistaken usage. There is a widespread belief that whenever IVN is used for less than 5 days, its instigation was some sort of misjudgement. Indeed, some experts have suggested that such 'misuse' of IVN is a valid audit criterion. This makes no sense. Although the concept that IVN is of no benefit to patients unless used for at least 5–10 days is derived from the results of some IVN trials, those results do not apply to normal practice since the studies were performed on patients who did not really need IVN support (see Chapter 3). Furthermore, in addition to IVN being discontinued as a result of a patient making good progress, IVN may also be discontinued early due to a complication such as loss of intravenous access (see Chapter 12). If an audit of the 'appropriate' use of IVN is required it should check on the validity of the indication for IVN at the time of its commencement and not on its duration (see Chapter 6).

Other relevant medical history and major organ function

Medical problems away from the gastrointestinal tract also influence the potential need for nutrition support and the best means of providing it. Your history must therefore establish whether there are significant problems affecting other systems, including:

- *Respiratory system*: could any respiratory problems have been caused by aspiration and/or would aspiration from oral intake or ETF pose a particular threat to the patient? Does the patient have respiratory failure which might be worsened by any overfeeding which can increase oxygen demands and carbon dioxide production (see Chapter 10)?
- *Cardiac function*: are there any cardiac problems which might be worsened by IVN, particularly the delivery of too much sodium and water? Have there been any cardiac rhythm problems that could be influenced by intravenous electrolyte administration (see Chapter 10)?
- *Liver function*: has there been any history of disordered liver function which might predispose to salt and water overload, infection, encephalopathy or bleeding risks from intravenous access or enteral tube placement (see Chapter 10)?
- *Pancreatic function*: is there any current or past history of pancreatic problems which might cause diabetes or malabsorption (strictly maldigestion) of oral or enteral feeds (see Chapter 10)?
- *Renal function*: is there any problem with renal function that may

cause abnormalities of fluid and electrolyte regulation (see Chapter 10)?

- *Neurological status*: is there any problem with diminished level of consciousness, restlessness, confusion or swallowing that will put the patient at risk of aspiration? Might neurological problems such as raised intracranial pressure lead to delayed gastric emptying?

Information on whether these systems are functioning normally will also be obtained from a review of the patient's laboratory results and your clinical examination.

Reviewing laboratory results

A review of the patient's recent haematological, biochemical and micro-biological results is an integral part of your assessment for nutrition support. The results affect decisions on both the most appropriate route of support and the regimen that should be provided. It is also important to have baseline blood results available before starting any IVN, so that you can recognise changes resulting from your intervention.

Although in most medical practice, laboratory information is reviewed after the findings on clinical examination, when assessing a referral for nutrition support, it is often better to be aware of any laboratory abnormalities and recent trends in results before going to see the patient. This helps you to identify and to some extent quantify the cause of the abnormalities that may have not been clear from the history. It will also guide your clinical examination, especially your interpret-ation of chart records relating to fluid balance. You also need the laboratory results, especially markers of organ function, when reviewing prescription charts.

Haematology

Haematology results contain a lot of important information, including the following:

- *Haemoglobin*: a deficiency of red blood cells (erythrocytes) and/or haemoglobin results in anaemia with symptoms including fatigue and shortness of breath. Causes are varied. Iron deficiency usually leads to a microcytic, hypochromic anaemia and results from lack of intake, poor absorption or excessive loss of iron (usually from bleeding). A macrocytic anaemia is usually due to poor intake or absorption of vitamin B_{12} or folic acid. Rarely, other nutritional deficiencies cause anaemia, usually in patients who have been malnourished or malabsorbing for prolonged periods, e.g. copper deficiency can cause a picture resembling iron deficiency.

- *White blood cell count (WBC)*: a high white blood cell count suggests the presence of infection. It is particularly used in IVN patients, in combination with the patient's temperature, general clinical status and inflammatory markers, to raise suspicion of catheter-related sepsis (CRS: see Chapter 12). If the WBC is low (a situation seen in oncology patients referred for IVN for their chemotherapy-induced gut damage), the patient will be very prone to infections and may not display the normal responses in terms of raised temperature. Such patients are therefore not only vulnerable to CRS but CRS or other infections can easily be missed. A low WBC therefore raises concerns in relation to instigating IVN and, although not an absolute contraindication, you will need to exercise particular caution.
- *Platelets*: low platelets usually indicate liver disease or bone marrow dysfunction including dysfunction due to drugs or nutrient deficiencies). They can also be destroyed by autoimmune processes. A low count will increase bleeding risks from placement of intravenous access.
- *Inflammatory markers*: raised C-reactive protein (CRP) or erythrocyte sedimentation rates (ESR) are markers of inflammation and, as with rising WBCs, suggest the possibility of CRS or other infections in IVN patients.

Biochemistry

As discussed above, decisions on starting IVN and the make-up of the regimen to be used cannot be made without knowing which organ systems are fully functional and the degree of impairment in those that are damaged. Furthermore, both starvation itself and the introduction of nutrition in malnourished individuals can precipitate serious biochemical abnormalities such as the refeeding syndrome (see Chapter 8). Biochemical assessments of the following are therefore vital:

- Sodium, potassium, urea and creatinine (which also provide information on fluid status and renal function)
- Magnesium, phosphate and calcium
- Liver function tests, including international normalised ratio (INR)
- Blood glucose

A summary of the important IVN prescribing considerations related to specific organ impairment is given in Chapter 10, with more details on the relevance and interpretation of serum biochemistry in Chapter 8. Biochemical measurements are of little or no value in determining cardiorespiratory function, although blood gas results and measures of lactate are valuable.

If a required biochemical measurement is missing, it can often be performed retrospectively on a recent sample (taken within the last 48 hours). This can be arranged by telephoning the laboratory, although magnesium and phosphate cannot usually be added because of time-dependent intracellular-to-extracellular leakage.

Microbiology

The results of any microbiological samples or cultures from your patient indicating the presence of infection may influence your decision on the need and best route for nutrition support, especially if they suggest CRS. The presence of infection may also influence nursing requirements such as the need to 'gown and glove' before carrying out your physical examination. Antibiotic prescriptions for any infection identified may affect fluid and electrolyte provision (see Chapter 5).

Clinical examination

Although results from a recent clinical examination of the patient are often available in the medical notes, it is important for you to conduct a brief assessment of your own to help you decide on the need for IVN and the best prescription of nutrients and fluids. The clinical examination should include assessment of:

- General and nutritional status
- Cardiorespiratory and fluid status
- Gastrointestinal status
- Neurological function
- Current and potential intravenous access

General examination and nutritional status

An 'end-of-bed' general assessment of patients gives an impression of their overall well-being as well as a preliminary assessment of nutritional, respiratory and neurological status. Patients' ability to move is an important consideration in assessing their longer-term energy needs.

An ideal examination of nutritional status includes proper measures of body weight and height, which are then compared with previously recorded measures or the patient's recollection. As mentioned above, however, both current and past weights and heights can be difficult to obtain and you are often limited to checking for the presence of any obvious muscle wasting and loss of subcutaneous fat, and looking for any signs of specific vitamin deficiencies. Appearances can be very deceptive in patients with any limb oedema (Plates 2a and 2b), which can make very thin arms and legs look quite robust. Pull up the patient's sleeve to get a more accurate picture of true upper-arm circumference.

Examination for signs of specific micronutrient depletion should include assessment of:

- *Mouth*: this is the one place that you can easily see the lining of the gastrointestinal tract and a ravaged, sore mouth suggests similar problems lower down. Even if it looks normal, ask patients if their mouth is sore and, assuming they have been allowed some oral intake, whether it is painful to eat or drink. Also ask whether food tastes normal, since some deficiencies, e.g. zinc, can cause loss or alteration of taste sensation. A red, sore tongue (Plate 3a) suggests B-group vitamin deficiencies, whereas a very smooth tongue (Plate 3b) may be due to iron deficiency. Poor iron status can also cause sores at each side of the mouth which hurt when eating or speaking (angular cheilitis). More generalised perioral sores, especially if the patient also has a perineal rash, suggest zinc depletion. Swollen, bleeding gums with loss of teeth occur in scurvy from vitamin C deficiency.
- *Hair*: recent abnormal hair loss or a change in hair growth towards finer, curly hair can follow any severe or chronic illness but is particularly seen in patients developing trace element deficiencies.
- *Skin*: specifically look for thinning of the skin, damage from minimal trauma and poor repair to such damage that occurs with malnutrition. Specific rashes or skin abnormalities can also indicate deficiencies such as zinc, vitamin C and some B-group vitamins (see Chapter 9). Dry, fragile, flaking skin can indicate essential fatty acid deficiency.
- *Nails*: periods of illness and poor nutrition lead to poor nail growth and nails that break easily. If these periods have been intermittent, the nails are sometimes horizontally ridged. Fragile, thin, spoon-shaped nails are another sign of iron deficiency.

Whilst performing the general clinical examination, you should also be looking out for loss of skin turgor, which suggests dehydration, or the presence of salt and water overload, which is manifest by general oedema (see below). You may also find signs suggestive of liver disease, including the presence of jaundice (look carefully at the whites of the eyes), white fingernails, red palms, thickening or contractures of finger flexor tendons in the palm (Dupuytren's contractures), breast enlargement in a male and spider naevi (red spots consisting of a central blood vessel that blanches if you press it, with radiating finer vessels – the 'spider's legs').

Cardiorespiratory and fluid status

Dehydration is suggested by loss of skin turgor, pale and cold extremities, a dry tongue, a dry oral mucosa and sunken eyes. You should also check on the temperature, pulse and respiration charts for tachycardia and hypotension. Even non-clinicians can learn to assess jugular venous pressure (JVP), which is usually low in dehydration. Your previous examination of the laboratory results (see above) and your examination of the fluid balance charts (see below) will help in your assessment. Rising urea and creatinine strongly suggest dehydration unless there is a specific problem affecting the kidneys and the diagnosis would be supported by negative fluid balance charts with falling urine outputs.

Fluid overload is suggested by the development of oedema and a raised JVP, especially if the patient is also breathless, with the shortness of breath made worse by lying flat (orthopnoea). As with dehydration, examination of laboratory results and the fluid charts also provides valuable clues. The development of hyponatraemia and high urine outputs will support your suspicion of fluid overload unless the patient has some types of chronic renal failure or is in the polyuric phase following acute renal damage.

Although non-medical professionals are not expected to examine the heart and lungs, it is important to be aware that fine crackles in the chest and added heart sounds can confirm fluid overload and/or cardiac failure, which will impact on decisions regarding fluid and electrolyte provision. Findings on respiratory examination suggesting aspiration may provide contraindications to continued oral and/or ETF.

Gastrointestinal tract

Examination of the gastrointestinal tract and abdomen is also largely beyond the remit of non-clinician IVN prescribers. However, a brief assessment of the abdomen, coupled with some questions to the patient and observations of outputs from tubes, stomas and drains, is useful. The presence of vomiting, high nasogastric tube aspirates and abdominal distension, along with the absence of bowel sounds or the passage of flatus/stool, are all indicators of a non-functioning gastrointestinal tract. They therefore suggest that oral intake or ETF will be poorly tolerated. Any abnormal losses will need to be considered in terms of type and volume when it comes to decisions on fluid, electrolyte and nutrient needs.

Neurological examination

A brief neurological assessment of level of consciousness, likely compliance with therapy, swallowing capacity and ability to feed is required. If the patient does have swallowing difficulties, the outcome of a speech and language therapy (SALT) assessment should be taken into account when considering the possibility and safety of offering any oral intake. The findings may also affect your recommendations regarding ETF.

Potential intravenous access

As discussed in Chapter 3, all IVN must be administered through dedicated intravenous feeding catheters. Your patient examination must therefore include assessment of any current intravenous access or whether suitable access is likely to be achievable.

Reviewing fluid balance, fluid prescription and nutrient intake charts

A review of fluid losses and both recent and planned fluid and nutrient intakes will enable you to consider IVN in the context of all other sources of support. You need to be aware, however, that the relevant charts are notoriously often incomplete, inaccurate or both. It is therefore particularly important to ask the patient and nursing staff whether anything may have been missed.

Fluid charts

The fluid charts are a source of information on your patient's fluid intake and losses. These intakes and losses can be by many different routes and

Table 4.1 Likely sources of fluid intake and loss

Sources of intake	Sources of loss*
Drinking	Urine output
Enteral feeds	Insensible losses (see text)
Intravenous nutrition	Surgical drain output
Intravenous fluids	Fistula output
Intravenous drugs	Gastric aspirates
Fluid through an enteral feeding tube	Vomiting
	Stool, especially via stomas or diarrhoea

* Fluid lost often contains significant quantities of electrolytes and other nutrients, e.g. small-bowel losses may contain large quantities of sodium and diarrhoea or stomal losses may contain large quantities of potassium and magnesium.

you must try to ensure that all are accounted for (Table 4.1). Fluid charts have a particular tendency to miss out intake from intravenous drugs and losses via drains, fistulae and the insensible route. The last consists of fluid evaporated from the lungs during respiration and losses from the skin via both direct transpiration and sweating. The total insensible loss depends on the clinical condition of your patient, especially the presence of pyrexia and the ambient temperature and humidity. It is often around 500–1000 mL/day or approximately 10 mL/kg per day.

The fluid volume that your patients need will vary greatly and you will therefore need to review their requirements at least daily to prevent unnecessary complications. Each review must include a brief clinical reassessment of their hydration status, reference to changes in laboratory results and a check on any IVN prescriptions, bearing in mind any overall aims in terms of achieving positive, negative or neutral fluid balance.

Intravenous fluid prescription charts

The intravenous fluid charts should tell you how much fluid has been given and what is planned for the immediate future. It is important to ensure that the fluid content of any IVN that you decide to give is fully accounted for to reduce the risks of fluid overload. A fluid prescription review also enables you to check what intravenous electrolytes have been given, particularly quantities of sodium and potassium. The amounts provided, coupled with any changes in recent daily laboratory results, can then guide your IVN prescribing.

For example, in a patient with renal impairment, the prescriptions for fluid and potassium over the last few days help your prescribing decisions when starting IVN. If the patient is clinically euhydrated and the charts show approximate fluid balance with a normal urine volume, you should simply continue with approximately the same quantity of fluid per day. Similarly, if potassium levels have been normal and stable with no intravenous potassium supplementation and little oral intake, the patient is likely to be retaining potassium and any additions to the IVN might cause hyperkalaemia. Conversely, if daily biochemistry checks show that potassium levels have been low or falling despite the patient receiving several grams of potassium chloride daily, the patient should have very generous potassium provision in the IVN.

Nutrient intake records

Food charts and enteral feeding prescriptions help with your assessment of recent and current nutritional intake and hence your determination of whether the patient can achieve adequate nutrition via oral or ETF means.

Food intake records

Food intake record charts should indicate what patients have been offered and, depending on the chart design, may also provide information on how much they actually consumed. Such charts should include nutritional supplements such as sip-feeds, although these should also be documented on the drug chart (see Chapter 5). However, food charts are often unreliable due to missed or inaccurate entries and you therefore need to follow them up by discussion with the patient and nursing staff. Always check any open sip-feeds on bedside tables and try to account for the nutritional value of any food consumed, bearing in mind whether they provide complete nutrition. For example, eating icecream may provide reasonable levels of energy and nitrogen but will not provide all micronutrients.

Enteral feeding prescriptions

Enteral feeding prescriptions give instructions for the administration of tube feeds to patients. Although not normally a 'prescription' in the legal sense, they should be viewed in the same light as drug prescriptions. A patient's tolerance to ETF is a useful marker of current gastrointestinal function. However, it is not uncommon for patients to receive much less than prescribed because of problems such as delays related to tubes being pulled out. You should therefore check the amount of feed given, look at the fluid balance chart and ask the patient and ward staff. It is also important to be clear whether a feeding tube is gastric or jejunal when interpreting tolerance. For example, concentrated feeds put directly into the jejunum rather than the stomach are more likely to cause diarrhoea. The type and position of feeding tubes are also important when considering their use for the administration of medicines (see Chapter 5).

Conclusion

Once you have completed your history, examination and assessment of food and fluid charts, you can decide whether nutrition support is needed and the best route to provide it. You will not, however, be able to prescribe safely unless you also assess the patient's current prescription charts (see next chapter).

5

Review of prescription charts

Introduction

Patients referred for intravenous nutrition (IVN) support tend to be complex, with most receiving many drugs. Most also have little or no capacity to take medications by mouth and will therefore need their drugs to be given intravenously or via enteral feeding tubes. It is therefore important that all prescription charts are assessed at the time of referral, not only to help in decisions on whether they require IVN and what should be given, but also to try to avoid interactions between IVN and other drugs, and any problems that might occur from providing other medication when routes of administration are restricted. The prescription chart review therefore aims to:

- Establish whether the patient's medications provide any additional clues to the nature and severity of other medical conditions
- Check for the possibility that IVN could not be avoided by reducing dosage or stopping any drugs that interfere with gut function
- Give a better understanding of gastrointestinal tolerance and determine the best routes available for drug administration
- Identify potential problems related to interactions between IVN and other intravenously administered drugs
- Avoid problems caused by drugs that may need to given via an enteral feeding tube
- Prescribe any nutrition support products or drugs that are needed instead of, or in addition to, IVN
- Identify whether any prescribed drugs will influence the content of a proposed IVN regimen
- Identify any relevant allergies, restrictions or sensitivities

The review should include 'once only' and 'as required' as well as the regular sections of the drug chart and should extend to include specialised prescription charts such as those used for cytotoxics or insulin.

Information on other medical conditions

Prescribed drugs and doses are useful indicators of the nature and severity of several medical conditions and, in some cases, a drugs review will identify clinical history that might otherwise have been missed. For example, pre-existing prescriptions for a diuretic and an angiotensin-converting enzyme (ACE) inhibitor suggest that the patient is prone to congestive cardiac failure and hence liable to develop fluid overload with IVN. Similarly, concurrent prescriptions for high-dose loperamide and codeine phosphate suggest that a patient who is unclear about a history of abdominal surgery has actually had extensive resection and may have a very short bowel (see Chapter 10).

Antibiotic or antifungal prescriptions on drug charts suggest that infection is suspected or confirmed (although they are occasionally used for prophylaxis). They should certainly prompt clarification of the reasons behind their prescription for not only can IVN worsen some infective processes but infections can also seed into intravenous catheters causing catheter-related sepsis (CRS: see Chapter 12). The apparent effectiveness of antibiotic prescriptions may also influence whether you commence IVN. It is inappropriate, for example, to start IVN in a patient with suspected CRS who remains pyrexial despite antibiotic therapy, while it may be reasonable to start IVN if all signs of CRS have resolved after 24–48 hours of appropriate therapy.

Drugs interfering with gut function

Many drugs affect gastrointestinal function and so can worsen intestinal failure or limit tolerance to enteral tube feeding (ETF). The most common examples are those that promote or cause ileus, including opioid analgesics and anticholinergics. These should therefore be reduced or stopped if possible whenever ileus underlies the IVN referral.

Many drugs also cause or exacerbate diarrhoea, which can also be the limiting factor in the effectiveness of ETF. Classes of drug causing this problem include histamine H_2-blockers, proton pump inhibitors, antibiotics, antiarrhythmics, antihypertensives and non-steroidal anti-inflammatory drugs. All laxatives should also be stopped if ETF appears to be causing loose stools and this includes medicines containing magnesium such as antacid preparations and those containing active fillers such as sorbitol.

Antibiotics can also cause diarrhoea and, although the problem is seen in patients eating normally, it is far more common in patients on

ETF. The exact reason for this is unclear but it seems likely that they alter intestinal flora and allow overgrowth of pathogenic species. *Clostridium difficile* toxin is found in 20–50% of patients with antibiotic-related diarrhoea[1]. Antibiotics also reduce colonic bacterial production of short-chain fatty acids from insoluble carbohydrates and fibre, and these normally help to maintain healthy colonic enterocyte function. Once again, if diarrhoea with ETF has precipitated the potential need for IVN, any antibiotics should be stopped or changed to a more specific agent if possible.

Gastrointestinal tolerance and best-prescribed routes for all drugs

Tolerance to, and the efficacy of, orally administered medicines gives some indication as to how well the gastrointestinal tract is working. For example, if whole capsules come out of a stoma, absorption must be poor and this is likely to apply to nutrients as well as drugs. Since many patients referred for IVN usually have difficulty with oral or even enteral tube-administered prescriptions, drug chart assessment should also consider the best routes to administer all medicines that the patient requires (Figure 5.1) and your review can also identify drugs that may be causing diarrhoea with oral or enteral nutrition (see Chapter 2).

If a drug cannot be given orally because of problems with swallowing or absorption, the following should be considered:

- *Give the drug by an alternative route*: clearly, many oral drugs can be given via an enteral tube (if a suitable formulation is available) or by the intravenous route. Dose changes may be needed (e.g. ciprofloxacin orally versus intravenously) and the change can also influence total fluid and electrolyte provision, e.g. many intravenous antibiotics are administered with significant quantities of sodium and water (see below).
- *Use an alternative drug formulation*: oral liquids or buccal preparations may be useful, although there may still be problems with some 'melt' formulations which, although dispersing in the mouth, are absorbed further down the gastrointestinal tract (check with manufacturer for specific drugs). Rectal or transcutaneous preparations can be effective.
- *Use an alternative drug.*
- *Do not give the drug*: if this option is taken, regular review of the need for, and potential to restart, the drug or use of an alternative will be required.

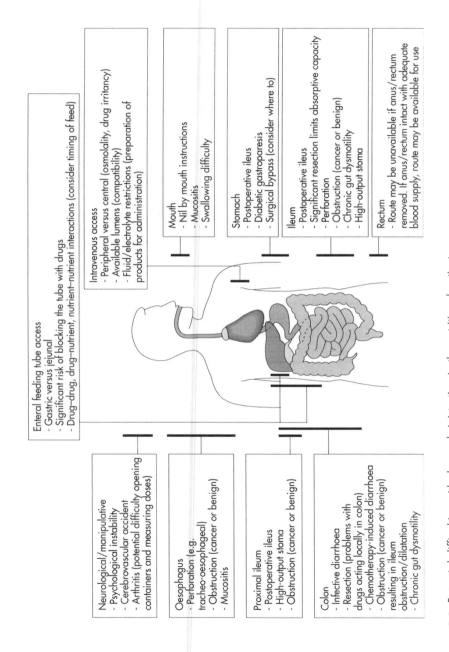

Figure 5.1 Potential difficulties with drug administration in the nutritional patient.

- *Incorporate drugs into your IVN regimen*: although it is possible to incorporate some drugs into IVN regimens, this usually creates risks (see Appendix 1).

If drugs do have to be given by alternative routes or are temporarily stopped, ensure that any amendments that are intended to be short-lived do not become permanent. Speech and language therapy (SALT) assessment of swallowing difficulties can be helpful.

Interactions between intravenous drugs and intravenous nutrition

If the intravenous route is to be used for feeding, potential interactions between drugs and the IVN will need to be avoided since they can reduce the efficacy of one or both prescriptions and may put the patient at serious risk. Different types of interaction include:

- *Antagonistic effects*: e.g. the presence of even small amounts of vitamin K in IVN lipids and/or vitamin K included in products such as Vitlipid Adult can make it difficult to achieve therapeutic levels of warfarin.
- *Precipitation of intravenous therapies*: precipitation of IVN with drugs administered through the same lumen can pose a serious risk of pulmonary embolus and line blockage, e.g. aciclovir[2].
- *Instability of IVN regimens due to dilution*: dilution of the lipid components of IVN will occur if other intravenous drugs or fluids are running through the same lumen. This can result in 'cracking' of the lipid and loss of emulsification (see Appendix 1). Dilution of the nitrogen component can also result in instability.
- *Instability of IVN regimens due to the presence of excessive electrolytes*: running additional electrolytes through the same lumen as the IVN can also result in lipid 'cracking' and emulsification loss (see Appendix 1). This includes the sodium content of a 0.9% w/v sodium chloride infusion.
- *Duplication of prescribing*: the administration of IVN containing micronutrients and electrolytes may lead to an excessive supply of these components unless other oral and/or enteral supplementation is stopped.

Avoiding problems from drugs given via enteral feeding tubes

Administration of medicines through an enteral feeding tube may seem to be the obvious choice when presented with a patient unable to take them by mouth but the practice should be avoided whenever possible since a number of problems can arise. Tube blockage occurs very easily if oral formulations are crushed and put down the tube and binding between drugs and enteral feed can occur either in the tube itself or in the upper gastrointestinal tract. For example, if preparations containing calcium, magnesium or phosphate are given at the same time as enteral feed, binding may result in reduced gut absorption. Ciprofloxacin[3,4] and phenytoin[5,6] also bind with enteral feeds. If there appears to be no alternative to the use of this route, the following questions need to be addressed:

- *Is this absolutely necessary?* Administration of the drug via the tube will almost certainly be unlicensed and the prescriber must be prepared to accept that responsibility.
- *Can the staff available undertake enteral tube administration of the drug safely?* Expertise is needed to ensure that drugs given via a tube are prepared in the correct dosage immediately prior to use, are not left unattended and are administered using enteral rather than parenteral syringes. Flushing must always be carried out using the largest syringe available to minimise the danger of the tube bursting from the pressure that can be generated.
- *Is the formulation appropriate?* Delayed or slow-release formulations (e.g. XL, SR drugs) cannot be crushed or opened without risk of inappropriate release of active ingredients, and potentially hazardous drugs, including some antibiotics, hormones, steroids and cytotoxics, cannot be crushed without risk to staff. Drugs with a narrow therapeutic index require careful monitoring for efficacy and toxicity when given via a tube. Blood monitoring of levels may be required.
- *Will the drug be tolerated?* Jejunal administration of irritant drugs or formulations can cause diarrhoea and hence limit effective absorption. Concentrated products may require dilution.
- *Will the drug block the tube?* Blockage of gastrostomy, jejunostomy or nasojejunal tubes causes significant problems and may be irreversible. 'Gloopy' liquids or formulations that are difficult to disperse are likely to block the tube, although dilution may be possible.

- *Is a change in formulation required?* Different formulations of the same drug may necessitate a change in dose, e.g. 90 mg of phenytoin suspension is equivalent to 100 mg of tablets or capsules[7].

- *What is the primary site of drug absorption?* If the primary site of absorption is above the jejunum, administration through a jejunal tube will be ineffective. 'Melt' formulations that dissolve in the mouth may be absorbed further down the gastrointestinal tract and so may or may not be effective (you need to check with the manufacturer). Surgical interventions may have altered anatomy and hence prevent absorption, e.g. orally administered drugs intended to act in the large bowel will not arrive there if the patient has a stoma.

- *Is concurrent enteral feed prescribed?* Enteral feeds interact with some drugs within the tube or gut if the time between feed and drug administration is inadequate and/or flushing is inadequate. For nasogastric administration, the feed should ideally be stopped for 2 hours before and 2 hours after the drug dose, although it is probably reasonable to reduce the time postdose to 1 hour if necessary. For jejunal administration, time between feed and drug can be reduced to 1 hour since prolonged jejunal pooling of drug or feed is less likely than in the stomach.

- *Are other drugs being put down the enteral tube?* Different drugs may also need separation from one other as well as from enteral feeds. Always flush the tube before and after each drug.

Specialist advice should be sought from a pharmacist when considering prescribing medicines to be administered through an enteral tube.

Prescribing nutrition support products and drugs related to intravenous nutrition

In some cases your clinical and nutritional review will lead to decisions to prescribe some nutritional supplements independent of any IVN. For example, you may wish to give thiamine supplementation to a patient at risk of Wernicke-Korsakoff syndrome, whatever the route of nutrient provision. A decision to start IVN may also lead to prescriptions other than for the IVN regimen itself. An example would be the use of glyceryl trinitrate patches to try to reduce the risk of peripheral vein thrombophlebitis (see Chapter 12).

The effects of all prescribed drugs on potential intravenous nutrition regimens

It is important to appreciate that many drug prescriptions or concurrent ETF will influence decisions on what to give in any IVN regimen. For example, many intravenous antibiotics contain large amounts of sodium (see below) and some drugs such as propofol, used for sedation, contain a lot of lipid calories[8] and may also affect distribution of lipid-soluble drugs. When considering any implications of intravenous drug administration on the IVN regimen, always remember to multiply the fluid and electrolyte load per dose by the frequency of administration, taking the diluent into account – see the Tazocin example in Chapter 8.

Other drugs promote electrolyte loss and hence create the need for greater IVN electrolyte provision, e.g. increased renal excretion of potassium with some diuretics[9] or potassium and magnesium loss with amphotericin B[10,11]. Amiloride may be used to reduce potassium losses induced by the use of amphotericin B[11].

Allergies, sensitivities and restrictions

Always check whether the 'allergies' box on drug charts contains any comments and be aware that the absence of information in the box does not necessarily mean that questions have been asked. For patients who really have no previously recognised problems, the box should state 'none known' and if the box is left blank you should seek relevant information from clinical notes, the patient, a previous prescription, the general practitioner or a relative or carer if absolutely necessary. For a patient with known problems, the effect that the drug responsible might have should be established in case giving that drug is clinically indicated and any risk has to be considered against the likely benefit.

IVN is suitable for most vegetarians but the lipid (see Chapter 7) may contain egg[12-14]. Vegans may therefore insist on lipid-free regimens and patients allergic to eggs should not be administered normal lipid products without supervision. Lipids based on soybean oil do not contain soya protein and hence can be used with caution in patients with soybean allergy[12].

Specialist prescription charts

In addition to the standard prescription charts, your patient may also have specialist charts that need review. Diabetic charts may be used to prescribe insulin and are often used to record results from blood glucose monitoring. Chemotherapy prescriptions are also written on separate specialist sheets in many settings and review will clarify the likely nature of any gastrointestinal damage such as mucositis, e.g. methotrexate frequently causes stomatitis if doses above 100 mg/m^2 are administered[15]. Cytotoxic drugs may result in increased electrolyte losses such as potassium and magnesium losses with the use of cisplatin[11].

Administration of intravenous drugs

Drugs prescribed for intravenous administration are not always given the same way each time they are prescribed. Although your choice of administration method will depend on local policy, alternative methods of administration may be required in some clinical situations. The use of a diluent other than either 5% w/v glucose or 0.9% w/v sodium chloride is rarely appropriate, although the use of small volumes of water for injection for reconstituting dry powders or as a diluent for bolus doses can sometimes be used. Your options may be restricted by stability, e.g. amphotericin must always be diluted in glucose, not sodium chloride, to avoid precipitation[16]. Further details are beyond the remit of this book.

References

1. Stroud M, Duncan H, Nightingale J. Guidelines for enteral feeding in adult hospital inpatients. *Gut* 2003; 52 (suppl. VII): vii1–vii12.
2. Trissel L. *Handbook on Injectable Drugs*, 13th edition. Bethesda: American Society of Health-System Pharmacists, 2005: 11.
3. Smyth J, ed. *The NEWT Guidelines for Administration of Medication to Patients with Enteral Feeding Tubes or Swallowing Difficulties*. Wrexham: North East Wales NHS Trust, 2006: 74.
4. Fair R, Proctor B. *Administering Medicines through Enteral Feeding Tubes*, 2nd edn. Belfast: Royal Hospitals, 2004: 56–57.
5. Smyth J, ed. *The NEWT Guidelines for Administration of Medication to Patients with Enteral Feeding Tubes or Swallowing Difficulties*. Wrexham: North East Wales NHS Trust, 2006: 188–189.
6. Fair R, Proctor B. *Administering Medicines through Enteral Feeding Tubes*, 2nd edn. Belfast: Royal Hospitals, 2004: 182–183.
7. British Medical Association and the Royal Pharmaceutical Society of Great Britain. *British National Formulary* 51. London: BMJ Publishing Group and RPS Publishing, 2006: 243–244.
8. AstraZeneca. Diprivan® (propofol) Injectable Emulsion. http://www. diprivan.com/sedation/clinical_questions.asp?shownav=sedation#question4 (accessed 11 June 2006).

9. Davies D, Ferner R, de Glanville H, eds. *Davies's Textbook of Adverse Drug Reactions*, 5th edn. London: Chapman and Hall, 1998: 459.
10. Dukes M, Aronson J, eds. *Meyler's Side Effects of Drugs*, 14th edn. Amsterdam: Elsevier Science, 2000: 922–925.
11. Davies D, Ferner R, de Glanville H, eds. *Davies's Textbook of Adverse Drug Reactions*, 5th edn. London: Chapman and Hall, 1998: 460.
12. Buchman A. *Handbook of Nutritional Support*. Pennsylvania: Williams and Wilkins, 1997: 33–34.
13. Pennington C. *Therapeutic Nutrition: A Practical Guide*. London: Chapman and Hall, 1988: 123.
14. Karran S, Alberti K, eds. *Practical Nutritional Support*. London: Pitman Medical, 1980: 107.
15. Allwood M, Stanley A, Wright P, eds. *The Cytotoxics Handbook*, 4th edn. Oxfordshire: Radcliffe Medical Press, 2002: 235.
16. Needle R, Sizer T, eds. *The CIVAS Handbook: The Centralised Intravenous Additive Services Reference*. London: Pharmaceutical Press, 1998: 67–68.

6

Decisions on intravenous nutrition

Introduction

Following your clinical assessment and review of all charts (see Chapters 4 and 5) you need to decide whether the patient requires nutrition support, the best means of providing it and what you are going to give (see Chapters 7–11). You also need to document your decisions (see below) and note any particular risks that may be involved (see Chapter 12).

Intravenous nutrition required

Some form of nutrition support should be considered in all patients who are either malnourished or at risk of malnutrition, as defined by the National Institute for Health and Clinical Excellence (NICE) criteria. These use body mass index, percentage weight loss and likely period without food intake (see Chapter 1). As previously discussed, however, giving intravenous nutrition (IVN) is not without risk and considerable cost and its use should therefore be reserved for patients that cannot be safely and adequately supported using either oral means or enteral tube feeding (ETF).

If IVN is indicated, it should be commenced as soon as practical to stabilise the patient and to prevent further decline. It should not, however, be commenced as an emergency, especially if this means starting patients on a regimen unsuitable for them. In particular, even if a patient is severely malnourished, IVN should never be started at night or over the weekend using a bag that has no electrolyte and micronutrient additions (see Chapter 16). Such out-of-hours commencement of IVN is usually something considered in the most malnourished patients, yet it is that group that are at greatest risk of refeeding problems (see Chapters 8 and 9). Commencing incomplete IVN could be fatal in such patients.

On first deciding that IVN is indicated, it is almost inevitable that you will have little idea as to how long it may be needed. In general terms, IVN should simply be continued for as long as is required or until a complication prevents its continued use. Certainly, it is totally inappropriate to continue IVN solely to reach some 'magic' number of days – something that can put a patient at unnecessary risk of complications. This practice appears to have arisen from so-called evidence that IVN given for less than 1 week is ineffective. That 'evidence' was derived from the well-known Veterans studies[1] in which IVN was used in an elective role in malnourished surgical patients. In many of the study subjects, however, other means of feeding could have been used and, indeed, the study protocol excluded all patients who had a definite need for IVN. Furthermore, IVN support was given at very high levels, which are now believed to cause complications. Many of the study results therefore have little or no relevance to current UK practice and in our experience it is not uncommon to see clear benefits from IVN within 24–72 hours of commencement. Furthermore, since those benefits sometimes include resumption of gastrointestinal function after a period of prolonged ileus, we not infrequently give IVN for 2–3 days but then find that we no longer need to. When this occurs, we do not feel that we were mistaken in starting the IVN since the patient's recovery of gastrointestinal function may not have occurred so promptly without it.

Planned, preset periods of IVN are sometimes used to improve a patient's general status for surgery or to see if they improve the status of a patient with very marginal gastrointestinal function, who has been slowly deteriorating and in whom malnutrition may now be further compromising appetite and absorptive capacity.

Any plans for long-term home IVN warrant very careful discussion. At the very least, home IVN takes several weeks to arrange as training is intensive and funding must be sought (see Chapter 1).

No intravenous nutrition required

There are a number of reasons why you might decide that a patient referred for IVN probably does not need it and overall, we tend to turn down 20–25% of our referrals. The most common reason for not immediately commencing IVN in a patient who has been referred is that, although NICE recommends *considering* IVN whenever oral intake or ETF is unable to meet a malnourished patient's needs (or the needs of patients at risk of malnutrition), in reality you often delay IVN commencement if you believe that there is a realistic chance that the patient will tolerate adequate oral or enteral nutrition within a day or two. However, if the patient then fails to make good progress, you must have a low threshold for commencing IVN.

Another common reason for deciding that IVN is not needed is that the patient could actually be fed by other means at the time of referral. This is usually by enteral tube if access can be obtained. However, if gaining such tube access is likely to be difficult and time-consuming, e.g. it will need radiological input that will take days to arrange, it is probably better to commence IVN while waiting to see if the efforts to gain enteral access are successful.

A dying patient would not usually be given IVN support but this is not always the case and discussions are needed with the patient's primary medical team.

Documenting your decisions

Whatever your plan for nutrition support, you will need to document your assessments in the patient's medical notes. You will also need to maintain notes for your own purposes, write all appropriate prescriptions and discuss your decisions with the patient's immediate care teams and pharmacy Technical Services (see Chapter 15).

The aims of your entries in the patient's medical notes are to ensure that:

- All care teams involved understand the reasons for your decisions and know your plans.
- All teams are made aware of any specific risks that your nutrition support might pose and how best to avoid them.
- There is a record of the decision-making process if this were to be required.

Clinical notes

Patients' clinical notes are their primary care document. They are read by various staff looking after the patient and sometimes (with appropriate permission) by patients themselves or their legal representative. Your entries must therefore be clear, unambiguous and professionally appropriate. Case notes easily become very extensive and so it is also important to try to keep your entries concise.

For most patients, you will make two types of entry in the notes. The first will be your assessment on referral, culminating in your decision to start or hold back IVN. The second will be a record of subsequent reviews to monitor the patient or to check that an original decision to withhold IVN is still appropriate.

First patient review

Your initial entry in the clinical notes should give a brief summary of your patient assessment (see Chapters 4 and 5). It will therefore comprise:

- *Patient information*: the patient's name, age, admission date and reason for admission.
- *Past medical history*: identifying issues relevant to the provision of nutrition support (e.g. diabetes or renal impairment).
- *Current inpatient history and reason for referral*: a summary of recent issues relevant to the provision of nutrition support.
- *The indication for IVN or the reason why its use is not necessary at present*: a summary statement of the patient's current needs for nutrition support and the best means of meeting them.
- *Brief details of the proposed regimen*: this will include the daily provision of the energy, nitrogen and fluid that will be provided (see Chapter 11) along with details on provision of any individual electrolytes or micronutrients that have the potential to cause problems, either because current levels are already high or low, or because clinical status makes it likely that they will become abnormal, e.g. renal failure or refeeding risk (see Chapters 8–10).
- *Objectives of giving IVN*: usually the support of the patient until IVN can be replaced by oral or enteral tube feeding.
- *Additional recommendations*: suggestions on any required access (e.g. a central line or nasojejunal tube), electrolyte supplementation, fluid provision, monitoring and drug changes.

Try to keep your entry relevant to the provision of nutrition support unless additional information is important. Carry out all the points in your plan that are your own responsibility and ensure that actions that you yourself will not be undertaking are going to be undertaken by appropriate staff. The time of day that you write in the clinical notes will affect the time at which different health staff read the entry. For example, documenting late in the day that a patient needs additional potassium in intravenous fluids is not likely to help unless you discuss things directly with the ward or cover team. If you carry out something that is usually someone else's responsibility, make it clear in the notes so that there is no duplication. If you have not made a full review but have only seen a patient briefly (usually to determine whether there is any likely need to start IVN that day), ensure that this is evident in the record so that no further request is made out of hours to the duty pharmacist (see Chapter 16).

Subsequent patient reviews

Records in the medical notes of subsequent patient reviews are almost always shorter than the initial entry. They should again focus on nutritional care, usually following a different format:

*   *Current clinical history*: how the patient is feeling, including issues such as appetite, nausea, abdominal pain or bloating and pain related to a midline catheter. Include a note of any complaints or symptoms that you are not expert in but which need attention from the patient's primary clinicians.
*   *Current clinical examination and relevant laboratory results*: specific information such as the presence of oedema, temperature, blood glucose and haematology/biochemistry results.
*   *Summary*: conclusions drawn from the above information, including the outcome of any discussions with other staff.
*   *Plan*: list numbered points that require action.

There is no need to duplicate all information from your previous days' entries unless there has been significant change.

Records of prescription

All drugs administered in hospital are related to a signed prescription or written order unless given by a clinician in an emergency. This policy should also apply to micronutrient supplements, oral sip-feeds, enteral feeding and IVN, even if local policy allows otherwise.

Oral supplements and enteral feeds

Careful prescription and administration records are needed for all oral and enteral supplementation in order to:

*   *Ensure that all patients and staff view nutrition supplements and enteral feeds as an integral part of treatment.*
*   *Ensure that all teams are aware of all nutrients given*: amounts provided and tolerance to oral and enteral nutrition may influence important clinical management decisions.

- *Minimise risks of interactions*: drug–drug, drug–nutrient and nutrient–nutrient interactions can significantly affect bioavailability and can block tubes (see Chapter 5).
- *Reduce risk of overdose*: excessive total nutrition supplementation can result in complications such as refeeding syndrome, particularly in those who are nutritionally depleted (see Chapters 8 and 9).
- *Record of administration*: the medicine chart provides a record of administration in case of future queries.

As with any drug, staff administering a nutritional therapy should sign the chart to say that it was given. A blank space can be left if it was not administered but it is better practice to enter a code explaining the reason for non-administration, e.g. 'patient refused', 'patient unable to take drug' or 'medicine unavailable'. Furthermore, a signature for administration does not necessarily mean the patient took an oral nutrient supplement provided or that it was effectively absorbed, since boxes are usually signed when patients are offered the supplement rather than when they have finished drinking it. Always ask the patient or ward staff whether supplements are being consumed, look at the fluid balance chart, and check any cartons left by the patient to see if they are full or empty. Remember that patients tend to overestimate their intake.

Intravenous nutrition prescribing records

All IVN prescriptions and records of administration are clearly an essential part of documentation. Detailed suggestions on this aspect of IVN provision are given in Chapter 11.

Endorsing prescription charts

The standard practice of the pharmacist endorsing charts in order to clarify prescriptions, supply medicines and to provide practical advice should be extended to include nutritional aspects of the various charts (see Chapter 5). Standard pharmacist endorsing is always important but it is also important to give specific consideration to the need for nutritional endorsing of prescription charts. Examples include:

- *Appropriate separation*: between incompatible drugs and oral or enteral feeds such as ciprofloxacin or phenytoin or anything containing a calcium, magnesium or phosphate salt.
- *Electrolyte salt forms* (Appendix 2): to show both the quantity

prescribed in units others may use and to identify any other electrolytes provided as a result of the salt used. For example, an intravenous phosphate infusion should be endorsed to show the precise salt to be used and the quantity of sodium and/or potassium as well as the phosphate in the volume of the salt and concentration used.

- *Dilution of oral sip supplements*: appropriate dilution may make them more palatable because they can be quite sweet to taste. Fresh water should be used for juice-type supplements and milk should be used for milky-type supplements.
- *Intravenous drugs*: include the fluid type and volume to be used as well as the electrolyte content (if any).

Nutrition team notes

In addition to all of the above, the nutrition team also need to keep their own notes which are used when medical notes are unavailable, e.g. the patient is off the ward, and for audit purposes (see Chapter 14). The nature and sophistication of nutrition team notes will vary with local needs, patient numbers and team composition. They need to be updated daily and ideally should include:

- *Nutrition summary*: including patient log number for audit purposes (see Chapter 14) as well as basic information, such as body mass index, recent weight loss and estimated initial energy requirements.
- *Clinical notes*: similar to the entries in the clinical notes but with additional information from other parts of the case notes, such as the results of imaging.
- A *haematology/biochemistry summary table*: essential for quick reference when reviewing the patient and for electrolyte prescription.
- A *summary of current patients and action points*.

Conclusion

Once the assessments described in Chapters 4 and 5 have been performed, the decision to provide IVN has been made and the documentation and communication outlined in this chapter are complete you will need to decide exactly what you are going to give them. This requires very careful consideration and is the subject of the next section of this book.

References

1. The Veterans Affairs Total Parenteral Nutrition Cooperative Study Group. Perioperative total parenteral nutrition in surgical patients. *N Engl J Med* 1991; 325: 525–532.

7

Fluid and macronutrient requirements

Introduction

The overall aim of nutrition support is to ensure that patients' total fluid and nutrient intakes meet all of their needs. These needs vary with nutritional status and the nature and complexity of their current condition. However, all patients will need a complete range of macro-nutrients including:

- Fluid
- Energy to fuel metabolic functions: this energy is predominantly derived from glucose and lipid (lipids are also the source of essential fatty acids)
- Nitrogen sources for the synthesis of protein and other elements required for tissue deposition, maintenance of function and the synthesis of transport proteins and immunoglobulins

Since both inadequate and excessive administration of fluid or macro-nutrients can be dangerous, this chapter discusses their requirements in detail. The need for electrolytes and micronutrients is covered in Chapters 8 and 9.

Fluid requirements

Careful consideration of fluid balance is important for all sick indi-viduals but is particularly important in most patients referred for intra-venous nutrition (IVN) since derangement of normal fluid intake, absorption and/or loss is almost inevitable whenever someone has intestinal failure or an inaccessible gastrointestinal tract. All routes of fluid gain and loss must be accounted for (see Chapter 4).

Estimating fluid volume needs

Fluid management is never as simple as the commonly heard rule that 'most patients require 3000 mL/day'. In order to calculate your patient's current fluid requirements, you should use Equation 7.1.

Fluid requirement = Measured losses + Insensible losses
– Adjustment for other necessary fluid intake
± Adjustment for overloaded or dehydrated patient   (Eqn 7.1)

The adjustments for fluid overload or dehydration in Equation 7.1 are made following a clinical examination of the patient and review of previous fluid charts (see Chapter 4). However, patients' fluid needs vary swiftly and you must therefore review them at least daily in order to prevent complications. Each review must include a brief reassessment of their hydration status.

Deciding on the type of fluid to give

The large number of fluids suitable for intravenous administration can be split into two major groups:

- *Crystalloids* contain salts (see Appendix 2), glucose or a combination of the two. The dissolved solutes are of very small size and so have marked effects on the osmolality of the fluid (below). The nature of the solutes will determine the effect on the patient. Excessive sodium provision, for example, will lead to complications such as hypernatraemia and/or oedema, whereas excessive glucose usage can lead to pseudohyponatraemia or true hyponatraemia if fluid-induced diuresis creates high sodium loss without matching intake.
- *Colloids* generally contain aqueous solutes of between[1] 0.5 micrometre and 1.0 nm. These are much larger than the solutes found in crystalloids. Colloids include plasma substitutes and expanders such as human albumin solution and starches. These products tend to have little specific role in the management of nutrition.

The most common crystalloid intravenous fluids used for slow infusion are 0.9% w/v sodium chloride, 5% w/v glucose and 0.18% w/v sodium chloride with 4% w/v glucose. Other more specialised fluids are available, such as Hartmann's, which is often used to replace intra-operative fluid losses.

Overzealous administration of intravenous fluids (particularly 0.9% w/v sodium chloride) is a common cause of fluid overload and oedema, although large volumes may be required in some patients with high gastrointestinal or renal fluid losses. A problem of iatrogenic over-administration of fluid that is particularly seen in IVN patients occurs when the patient continues to receive inappropriate saline infusions despite commencement of an IVN regimen which also contains sodium and water. You must therefore be sure to discuss the ongoing plans for total fluid administration from IVN and all other sources with the clinical teams involved in any IVN patient's care.

The presence of oedema is of particular importance in IVN patients since it is often accompanied by oedema of the gut wall. This limits absorptive capacity and can cause or prolong ileus. However, it is important to recognise that oedema in patients can result from their illness *per se*, especially from recent surgery or sepsis. These insults result in extravasation of fluid from the intravenous compartment into the third space and this takes time to resolve. During this period, you should aim to provide enough fluid to maintain intravascular volume but try to ensure that you do not exacerbate fluid retention. Further administration of sodium should be particularly restricted in most such cases. Random urinary sodium measurements may be helpful (see Chapter 8).

The use of 5% w/v glucose infusions in vulnerable individuals can induce the refeeding syndrome (see Chapters 8 and 9). Specific fluids may be required for the administration of a stable dilution of drugs, for example, amphotericin must only be diluted in 5% w/v glucose and not 0.9% w/v sodium chloride in order to prevent precipitation[2].

It is important to take into account the volume of IVN in relation to any fluid restriction or other fluids the patient is receiving in order to achieve the correct volume of fluid and quantity of solutes for your individual patient. You must therefore be aware of all routes and types of fluid intake when deciding upon fluids within the IVN regimen. You should also aim to incorporate supplemental intravenous fluids into your IVN prescribing where practical (see Chapters 4 and 11).

Fluid osmolality issues

Fluid osmolality describes the osmotic pressure of a solution and is measured in milliosmoles (mOsm) per kilogram of solution (for common crystalloid fluids this is abbreviated to mOsm/kg water). The measure differs from osmolarity, which refers to the number of mOsm per litre of solution.

Table 7.1 Components and concentration of common intravenous fluids

Intravenous fluid	Approximate contents per 1000 mL (all in water for injection)	Approximate concentration (mOsm/kg water)*
0.9% w/v sodium chloride ('normal saline')	154 mmol sodium and 154 mmol chloride	300
5% w/v glucose	50 grams glucose	300
0.18% sodium chloride with 4% w/v glucose	30 mmol sodium, 30 mmol chloride and 40 grams glucose	300
0.9% w/v sodium chloride with 2 grams potassium chloride	154 mmol sodium, 154 mmol chloride, 27 mmol potassium	332
0.9% w/v sodium chloride with 3 grams potassium chloride	154 mmol sodium, 154 mmol chloride, 40 mmol potassium	360
Typical intravenous nutrition regimens	Very variable	Commonly > 900

* Normal plasma osmolality is 280–295 mOsm/kg water

The usual osmolality of plasma is 280–295 mOsm/kg water and fluids of a lower concentration are described as hypotonic whereas fluids of higher concentration are hypertonic (irrespective of the type of solutes in the fluid). The intravenous administration of large volumes of either hypotonic or hypertonic fluids invariably leads to complications. Hypotonic fluids can cause cell haemolysis whereas hypertonic fluids can cause cell dehydration or crenation. In addition, the more hypertonic an infusion, the more likely it is to cause venous thrombophlebitis (see Chapter 12).

The solutes in commonly used crystalloid intravenous fluids contribute to the overall osmolality of the solution (Table 7.1). IVN, which inevitably contains large amounts of additional components, is always very hypertonic, with typical osmolalities of > 900 mOsm/kg water.

The maximum recommended concentrations for peripheral administration of IVN are usually around 900 mOsm/kg water, since higher concentrations tend to cause thrombophlebitis. However, you have to differentiate between administration via a peripheral cannula into a very small vein compared to administration via a midline-type catheter which delivers IVN into larger upper-limb veins (see Chapter 3). This can often tolerate the higher concentrations of IVN usually administered centrally rather than peripherally[3].

Fluid used in intravenous nutrition formulation

Fluid in an IVN regimen can be prescribed in many different ways and your choice of components will partly be based on your patient's fluid requirements. For example, the availability of glucose in a variety of concentrations gives you flexibility since 500 mL of 20% w/v glucose provides the same energy as 1000 mL of 10% w/v glucose but in half the volume (see Appendix 2).

If you are using precompounded and sterilised triple-chamber IVN bags (see Chapter 11), you will have fewer options. Nevertheless, you can administer part bags or give a complete bag over a different time period (never more than 48 hours and subject to stability). You may also be able to add 0.9% w/v sodium chloride to some precompounded regimens, although stability would first need to be confirmed with the manufacturer. More details on IVN stability can be found in Appendix 1.

Levels of energy provision

For the purposes of this book, we refer to kilocalories (kcal) as the units for measurement of energy. 1 kcal is the amount of energy required to raise the temperature of 1 kg of water by 1°C. Energy can also be expressed in kilojoules (kJ) and an approximate conversion between the two is shown in Equation 7.2[4].

1 kcal = 4.2 kJ (approx.)   (Eqn 7.2)

Estimating energy requirements

The calculation of both energy and nitrogen needs is usually based around equations that account for the following factors:

- Patients' weight, age and sex
- Likely stresses imposed by their illness
- Current activity levels
- The stimulus to metabolism of giving the food itself (the thermic effect of feeding)
- Unusual fluid or nutrient losses
- Any need to make up nutrient deficits

Body weight can sometimes be obtained from a recent entry in medical notes, nursing records or an anaesthetic chart but if no measurement is available you will need to try to arrange for the patient to be weighed. This is not always possible and you may have to depend on the patient's

Table 7.2 Estimated daily basal metabolic rate from 1985 Schofield equations*

Years of age	Male	Female
15–18	(17.6 × (wt)) + 656	(13.3 × (wt)) + 690
19–30	(15.0 × (wt)) + 690	(14.8 × (wt)) + 485
31–60	(11.4 × (wt)) + 870	(8.1 × (wt)) + 842
60 plus	(11.7 × (wt)) + 585	(9.0 × (wt)) + 656

(wt), patient's weight in kilograms.

* These equations have since been updated but the initial versions have proved practically useful.

recollection, an estimate from a close relative or carer, or any estimate that you make yourself. Measured weights need to be adjusted for likely dehydration which can easily lead to underestimates of 1–2 kg, or fluid overload which, with oedema and/or ascites present, can cause over-estimates of 10, 20 or even 30 kg or more (see Chapter 4).

Patients' body weight, age and sex are initially used to estimate basal metabolic rate (BMR – resting energy expenditure when starved and undertaking no activities) from standard equations such as those of Schofield (Table 7.2) or Harris and Benedict. However, BMR can also be measured at the bedside using an indirect calorimeter – an instrument that calculates resting metabolic rate (RMR) from the patient's oxygen consumption and carbon dioxide production. RMR is equal to BMR if the patient is starved and lying still at the time of measurement. Indirect calorimetry can be very useful in a complex patient but the technique requires time and specialist equipment and is not widely available.

Obese patients have relatively more fat cells than the non-obese and so have fewer metabolically active cells per kg body weight. The Schofield equations therefore tend to overestimate the BMRs of heavy patients. Conversely, very thin patients with little fat have relatively greater metabolically active tissues per kg body weight and hence BMR estimates tend to be low.

Any activity increases energy requirements above BMR, as do changes in metabolism with illness, pyrexia and the metabolic stimula-tion of feeding itself. For this reason, estimates of actual energy require-ments are often made by adjusting the estimates of BMR to account for activity, stress and feeding factors. Adjustments are also suggested to provide for weight gain or weight loss if desirable. The most commonly advocated adjustments are shown in Table 7.3.

Table 7.3 Commonly recommended adjustments to basal metabolic rate (BMR) to allow for stress factors, activity and feeding effects

Type of factor	Examples	Modification to BMR
Metabolic stresses	Per degree pyrexia > 37°C	+10%
	Long-bone fracture	+10%
	Moderate infection	+10%
	Postoperative	+10%
	Chronic sepsis	+10%
	Inflammatory bowel disease	+10%
	Severe infection	+20–30%
Activity levels	Unconscious	No modification
	Awake but bed-bound and immobile	+10%
	Bed-bound and mobile or sitting	+15–20%
	Mobile on ward	+25%
	Ventilated and paralysed	−15%
Metabolic effect of feeding	Patient on intravenous nutrition	+10%
Desired weight change	Weight gain	+600 kcal
	Weight loss	−600 kcal

Concerns regarding estimated energy requirements

The use of the activity, stress and feeding factors shown in Table 7.3 and added to BMR leads to the apparent need for sicker patients to receive very large quantities of energy, especially if they are already nutritionally depleted (which is often the case for patients requiring IVN support). However, although the metabolic requirements of sicker patients may be high, they often diminish quite quickly[5] and, since net catabolism in such sick patients cannot be stopped, they also receive a considerable nutrient supply from the breakdown of their own tissues. They are therefore at potential risk of overfeeding problems. Many authorities have therefore concluded that such high levels of energy provision should specifically be avoided in the more seriously ill patient group, citing in support observations including:

- Feeding at levels above actual requirements (widely advocated during the early development of IVN) had definite adverse effects on clinical outcome[6].

- Providing high levels of energy may induce refeeding syndrome or other refeeding complications (see Chapters 8 and 9).
- Sick and/or malnourished patients are likely to have an increased requirement for micronutrients (e.g. to support wound healing) as well as having an existing deficiency. High levels of macronutrients cannot be utilised properly in the presence of such deficiency. Indeed, excessive macronutrient provision may deplete micronutrient stores even further and so create acute, threatening clinical deficiency such as that seen in Wernicke–Korsakoff syndrome (see Chapter 9).
- Most trials showing benefit from short-term nutrition support do so despite 'too little nutrition' being given for 'too short a time' for the benefit to accrue from maintaining or improving body energy and protein stores[7].
- Higher levels of feeding increase oxygen consumption and carbon dioxide production and so may worsen respiratory failure.
- Severely ill patients are often insulin-resistant and so high levels of feeding will produce relative hyperglycaemia (a particular concern, since a large intensive care trial demonstrated outcome benefits from tight blood glucose control[8]).
- A study of outcomes in intensive care patients showed that survival was best among patients receiving 33–66% of their estimated nutrient needs compared to those receiving either < 33% or > 66%[9].

Recommended energy provision

In the light of the above concerns, we suggest that the initial aim for energy provision in all cases should be based on BMR as estimated from a Schofield-type approach plus 20%. However, we also suggest that, in more severely ill or injured patients, nutrition support is only started at 50% of these calculated needs or even less if there is an extreme risk of refeeding syndrome (see Chapter 8). Full provision of fluid, electrolytes and micronutrients is required from the outset in all patients. Once patients are established on feeding and stable, energy provision can be increased to meet their full estimated requirements or even to exceed them if they have lost a lot of weight and replenishment is indicated.

The practices recommended above are in line with those recommended by the National Institute for Health and Clinical Excellence (NICE) in terms of generally cautious levels of energy provision with up to 50% introductory rates for the more seriously ill. The NICE

Box 7.1 National Institute for Health and Clinical Excellence (NICE) recommendations on macronutrient provision[6]

For patients who are not severely ill or injured or at risk of refeeding syndrome, the suggested nutritional prescription for total intake (from any food, oral fluid, oral nutritional supplements, enteral feeds and intravenous fluid/intravenous nutrition) should provide:

- 25–35 kcal/kg per day total energy (including that derived from protein)
- 0.8–1.5 g protein (0.13–0.24 g nitrogen)/kg per day
- 30–35 mL fluid/kg (with allowance for extra losses from drains, fistulae, etc. and extra input from other sources, for example, intravenous drugs)
- Adequate electrolytes, minerals and micronutrients to meet the patient's needs, taking into account any pre-existing deficits, excessive losses or increased demands

Seriously ill or injured patients requiring enteral or intravenous nutrition support should have feeding introduced cautiously at approximately 50% of estimated final target energy and protein requirements, building up to meet their full needs over the first 24–48 hours according to metabolic and gastrointestinal tolerance. Full requirements of fluid, electrolytes, vitamins and minerals should be provided from the outset of feeding

guidelines, however, recommend energy provision based more simply on body weight rather than estimates based on BMR with a percentage increment or stress factors added. Their recommendation of 20–30 kcal/kg per day is shown in Box 7.1, along with some of their other recommendations pertinent to fluid, energy and nitrogen provision. Their additional recommendations on the very cautious provision needed for patients at high risk of refeeding syndrome are contained in Chapter 8.

Meeting a patient's energy needs

The energy contained in IVN regimens comes in the form of glucose, lipid and nitrogen and the proportions provided by each need to be appropriately balanced.

Energy from glucose

Glucose provides 4 kcal/g and is generally a readily available energy source but it does require adequate endogenous or exogenous insulin for cellular uptake and there has been considerable debate regarding the

Table 7.4 Energy provided from different glucose concentrations*

Concentration	Volume (mL)	Energy (kcal)	Notes
5% w/v	500	100	Approximately isotonic
10% w/v	500	200	Hypertonic
20% w/v	500	400	Hypertonic
30% w/v	500	600	Hypertonic
40% w/v	500	800	Hypertonic
50% w/v	500	1000	Hypertonic
70% w/v	500	1400	Hypertonic

* 500 ml volume is used for consistency but different volumes may be available at each concentration. Doubling the volume provides double the energy for a fixed concentration.

maximum rates at which patients can utilize glucose, particularly when critically ill[10]. Current thinking, however, suggests that maximal glucose oxidation rates are not much affected by critical illness, remaining at around 4 mg/kg free fat mass/min[11]. This equates to around 800 kcal/day for a thin 40-kg patient with 10% body fat and 1600 kcal/day for a larger 90-kg patient with 20% body fat. These levels are not therefore likely to be exceeded if our recommendations to commence feeding cautiously in the critically ill are followed (see above) and furthermore, the ability to store excess glucose as either glycogen or (after conversion) as lipid will potentially accommodate provision at up to twice these utilisation rates as long as enough insulin is provided[11].

Excessive provision without adequate insulin will of course result in hyperglycaemia, especially in patients with insulin resistance, which includes most of the critically ill. This may then be associated with other complications such as infection (see Chapter 12). It is therefore usual practice to commence sliding-scale insulin in response to IVN-induced hyperglycaemia rather than restricting the IVN glucose content (see below). The incorporation of insulin into IVN regimens is considered in Appendix 1.

Glucose is available in a wide range of concentrations (Table 7.4). This is helpful when you are designing regimens from individual components (see Chapter 11) since it allows you to tailor the regimen towards a particular final volume by using or diluting higher strengths.

Glucose significantly increases IVN osmolality and so lipid-free regimens, which inevitably have high glucose levels to meet energy needs, should not be infused through peripheral cannulae or midlines since they are likely to cause thrombophlebitis.

Table 7.5 Typical energy provided from different lipid concentrations

Concentration	Volume (mL)	Energy (kcal)	Notes
10% w/v	500	550	Other volumes available
20% w/v	500	1000	Other volumes available
30% w/v	333	1000	No other volume available

Energy from lipid

Lipid provides 9 kcal/g regardless of the type or brand. It will therefore provide the same energy per unit volume for a given concentration (Table 7.5).

The use of lipid in IVN regimens has several advantages:

- *Source of essential fatty acids*: the essential fatty acids within lipid have many important functions beyond the simple provision of an energy source. These include the maintenance of cell membrane structure and function and the modulation of immune and inflammatory responses.
- *Concentrated energy source*: lipid helps in the formulation of lower-volume IVN regimens than those of the same total energy compounded using glucose alone.
- *Low osmolality compared to glucose*: lipid is particularly useful in regimens administered peripherally since the same energy level can be met with a lower-osmolality feed than feeds made using glucose as the sole energy source.

Lipids used in IVN regimens are mainly triglycerides, which consist of three fatty acids attached to a glycerol backbone (Figure 7.1). The fatty acids consist of carbon chains of various lengths that may contain one or more double bonds. The location of the first double bond in the chain is indicated by either the symbol ω (omega) or the letter n.

There are two essential fatty acids: ω_6-linoleic acid and ω_3-linolenic acid. Deficiency results in dermatitis, reduction in growth, diarrhoea, fatty liver, abnormal platelet function, hair loss and impaired wound healing[12–14].

The balance of IVN provision of ω_6-linoleic acid versus ω_3-linolenic acid is also of potential importance. ω_6-Linoleic acid is converted to arachidonic acid, which is incorporated into cell membranes and metabolised to proinflammatory prostaglandins and leukotrienes (e.g. prostaglandin E_2). This can theoretically result in adverse effects such as

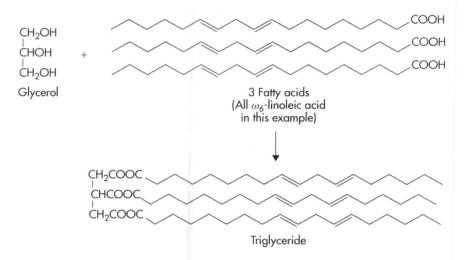

Figure 7.1 Triglyceride formation from individual fatty acids and glycerol.

platelet aggregation, inflammation, increased vascular permeability, fever and impairment of immune function. ω_3-Linolenic acid, on the other hand, is converted to eicosapentaenoic acid and docosapentaenoic acid, which are also incorporated into cell membranes. The arachadonic acid content is therefore reduced and subsequent metabolism produces less inflammatory prostaglandins and leukotrienes.

It has been recommended that 2–4% of total calories be provided as ω_6-linoleic acid in order to prevent essential fatty acid deficiency[12,13] but traditionally IVN lipids have a much higher content which may have adverse effects. Newer lipid sources seek to remedy this and other potential problems (see below).

Energy from nitrogen sources

The nitrogen provided in IVN as amino acids (AAs) is also used for energy, yielding approximately 4 kcal/g protein. Commercial preparations of IVN AAs are available in different strengths but commonly contain either 9 or 14 g nitrogen/litre, yielding approximately 250 and 350 kcal/litre respectively. In the past, it was accepted practice to exclude this energy derived from protein from estimates of the overall energy provided by IVN regimens when planning to meet a patient's demands. Behind this practice was the concept that all the nitrogen content of the IVN would be needed for tissue maintenance and repair and hence it would not be available for oxidation and energy production. However, this is completely incorrect unless the patient is in a state of dramatic net anabolism, which is unusual, if not impossible, in IVN patients. Indeed, the vast majority of IVN patients are catabolic to some extent, in which case the overall oxidation of nitrogenous compounds (mainly protein) must exceed the total that the IVN supplies. The net energy delivery from nitrogen will therefore exceed that in your IVN in nearly all cases.

In view of the above, it is essential that you are always absolutely clear whether the total energy quoted for an IVN regimen includes that from nitrogen or is referring to non-nitrogen energy, since the nitrogen component adds around 5 kcal/kg per day depending on the patient and the formulation. If this additional energy provision is not accounted for, you will risk giving too much with possible adverse consequences. Furthermore, some authorities believe that the overprovision of nitrogen itself, especially as free AAs, can have detrimental effects in sick patients (see below).

Nitrogen for non-energy purposes

In addition to its role in providing energy, the nitrogen content of IVN is essential in providing the building blocks, i.e. AAs used for lean tissue maintenance and growth, and the production of plasma transport proteins and the proteins involved in inflammation, immunity and repair.

Nitrogen is usually provided in IVN regimens as free AAs but the specific AA content varies with brand and the individual product that you are using. You can convert between nitrogen and protein content using Equation 7.3.

1 g nitrogen = 6.25 g protein (Eqn 7.3)

When prescribing nitrogen in IVN regimens, you need to consider the patient's estimated nitrogen requirements, the ratio of nitrogen to non-nitrogen energy in the regimen (see below) and any specific AAs that may be beneficial (see below). These considerations must be accommodated within your overall IVN prescription, keeping within constraints imposed by the range of standard, precompounded and sterilised triple-chamber bags that you keep (see Chapter 11) and/or your local compounding facilities (see Chapter 15).

Estimating nitrogen requirements

In healthy individuals, a protein intake equivalent to < 0.15 g nitrogen/kg per day is adequate to maintain nitrogen balance but this changes dramatically in acute illness since catabolic patients have very high nitrogen losses. In the past, this led to recommendations that feeds containing very high levels of nitrogen should be given to patients who were very ill or undernourished but recent thinking suggests this may be unwise. Observations behind such thinking include:

- Studies show that higher levels of protein provision (e.g. 0.25 g nitrogen/kg per day) reduce net lean tissue loss but do not grant improved clinical outcomes. Studies of even greater levels of provision (e.g. 0.3 g nitrogen/kg per day) do not yield additional lean tissue-sparing[6].
- The AAs needed for synthesis of acute-phase proteins differ from those needed for the more 'normal' synthesis of structural and transport proteins[15] and the pattern required does not match that provided by either food or commercially available nutrition support products. Excess nitrogen provision from standard products may therefore result in excess free AAs, which may have detrimental effects unless they are oxidised or metabolism is diverted away from acute-phase protein production towards the more 'normal' pathways.
- Excessive protein administration can lead to net fluid loss in order to support the excretion of unwanted nitrogen. This can then produce dehydration[16].
- High-protein and or/high-energy feeding has been shown to increase mortality in animal models of sepsis[17].
- The mortality of very malnourished, oedematous, severely ill adults in refeeding camps following famine appears to be increased by high-protein provision compared to those receiving low-protein diets[18], as has that of children[19].

In view of these observations, we recommend initial target intakes of around 0.15 g nitrogen/kg per day, i.e. close to those required for normal minimum maintenance. NICE also recommends a similar, lower-nitrogen approach, suggesting initial target levels of 0.13–0.24 g nitrogen/kg per day (Box 7.1). Nevertheless, some authorities are still convinced that higher levels of nitrogen provision should be given to more catabolic patients[20] and still recommend feeding at levels of 0.2–0.3 g nitrogen/kg per day.

Table 7.6 Advantages and disadvantages of using glucose and lipid as energy sources in intravenous nutrition regimens

Energy source	Potential advantages	Potential disadvantages
Glucose	• Readily usable energy source (in the presence of insulin) • Low cost • Different concentrations can be used to adjust towards desired volume	• Hyperglycaemia • High osmolality • High concentrations may compromise hepatic function
Lipid	• Provides essential fatty acids • Energy-dense (high energy in low volume) • Low osmolality • Allows for more efficient use of amino acids than using glucose alone	• Stability, particularly in high-volume, relatively low-lipid regimens • May result in hyperlipidaemia, affecting different lipid fractions with potential increase in atheroma risks • May compromise macrophage function and resistance to infection • Large amounts likely to compromise hepatic function in longer term

Balancing macronutrient provision

Once you have determined your patient's total energy and nitrogen needs, you must decide upon the relative ratios of each of the macronutrients within your planned regimen. It is simplest to begin with the nitrogen component which, as already discussed, is simply decided on the basis of body weight. The energy content from the nitrogen you are to give can then be subtracted from the total estimated energy target, leaving that which you must provide from glucose and lipid. In most cases, provision of this remaining energy should then be given from glucose and lipid in a ratio of around 50:50, so that you obtain advantages from each whilst minimising any disadvantages (Table 7.6).

A ratio of 60:40 in favour of either the glucose or lipid is acceptable, although it is probably better to favour a higher glucose level if you have the choice (unless osmolality is important because of peripheral administration). Calculating this ratio excludes the nitrogen energy, as shown in the examples given in Table 7.7.

Table 7.7 Calculating glucose to lipid energy ratios in intravenous nutrition regimens

Example	Nitrogen (kcal)	Glucose (kcal)	Lipid (kcal)	Total energy (kcal)	Glucose:lipid ratio (% glucose)
1	350	1400	550	2300	72
2	350	1000	1000	2350	50
3	250	600	550	1400	52
4	250	1000	0	1250	100

All lipid-free IVN regimens have a glucose-to-lipid ratio of 100:0, which is far from ideal. However, lipid-free regimens are used in some circumstances, including patient hypersensitivity to IVN lipids, and attempts to protect hepatic function (see Chapter 12) and line patency in long-term home IVN patients.

Non-nitrogen energy to nitrogen ratio

In addition to considering glucose-to-lipid ratios, you should also ensure that your non-nitrogen energy-to-nitrogen ratio is within an appropriate range. This will allow optimal utilisation of the nitrogen provided by minimising unnecessary oxidation of AAs (Equation 7.4).

Non-nitrogen energy (kcal) per gram of nitrogen
in IVN regimen = 150–250   (Eqn 7.4)

Recommendations for the exact ratio to aim for in Equation 7.4 vary considerably but it is unlikely that the precise value is critical. Furthermore, you will probably be restricted in your choice of ratio by the availability of precompounded and sterilised triple-chamber IVN bags (see Chapter 11). When this does occur, you should base your intended regimen on the patient's estimated energy requirements, ensuring any bag that you do prescribe has a reasonable nitrogen-to-energy ratio. Patients on longer-term IVN require an increase in nitrogen provision when energy provision is increased so that an appropriate balance between components is maintained.

Starting intravenous nutrition feeding

As discussed above, we believe that it is best to start all IVN cautiously to minimise risks of refeeding syndrome and to ensure that you do not

Table 7.8 Energy rate examples for intravenous nutrition (IVN) feeding

Approximate estimate of daily energy requirements	IVN volume containing estimated energy requirements	Full-rate feeding	Half-rate feeding	Quarter-rate feeding
1700 kcal	2000 mL	83 mL/hour (= 2000 mL/24 hours)	42 mL/hour	21 mL/hour
1200 kcal	2000 mL	83 mL/hour (= 2000 mL/24 hours)	42 mL/hour	21 mL/hour
2200 kcal	1500 mL	63 mL/hour (= 1500 mL/24 hours)	32 mL/hour	16 mL/hour

deliver excessive macronutrients without adequate micronutrients and electrolytes, especially when starvation or stress has diverted metabolism from its usual pathways. The same approach is also recommended by NICE (Box 7.1). To achieve this, we suggest that you consider IVN in terms of full-rate, half-rate and quarter-rate administration, where full-rate refers to provision of nutrition over 24 hours at a level that would meet your estimation of patients' initial energy needs, i.e. BMR + 20% in most cases. Half-rates can then be used as the starting level for the first 24–48 hours for most patients, with quarter-rates used in patients at very high risk of refeeding problems (see Chapters 8 and 9). Some examples are shown in Table 7.8. It is important to note, however, that the aim is to provide 50% or 25% of energy and protein needs during early cautious feeding but to meet 100% of likely fluid, electrolyte and micronutrient needs (see Box 7.1). Additional intravenous fluids are therefore required in most cases and the IVN bags prepared for administration at half-rate or quarter-rate will need twice or four times the estimated daily electrolyte and micronutrient content in order to meet patients' daily needs (see Chapters 8 and 9).

Continuing intravenous nutrition feeding

Once full-rate IVN is established, it probably takes most patients 10 days or more to become metabolically stable and replete in micronutrients, especially if they were significantly malnourished and/or very ill at the time of IVN commencement. Improved gastrointestinal function allows many patients to come off IVN during this period but, for those who need to continue, changes will need to be made.

Once stability is achieved, energy and nitrogen provision should be adjusted to meet longer-term needs or to replete pre-IVN deficits. Any increase should usually be made in steps, increasing provision by 200–400 kcal/day, every 2–5 days. Monitoring to ensure tolerance should be made before each step-up, using factors including overall clinical condition, biochemical stability, hepatic function, oedema and changes in weight. If aiming for weight change, plan for gradual alteration and remember any rapid change is likely to be due to fluid rather than tissue.

In addition to changes in energy and nitrogen provision you should also consider increasing the rate of feeding to give a feed-free break for a few hours in every 24 hours for patients who are likely to continue IVN for several weeks. This is achieved by giving the same nutrients and volume of IVN per 24-hour period but providing it over a shorter duration at a faster rate. This then allows the patient more freedom and the physiological break in feed delivery may help limit IVN-induced liver damage in the longer term (see Chapter 12). A gradual increase in rate is necessary, reducing the duration by 4 hours each time and allowing several days at each step to ensure tolerance at that level before continuing to the next. Be careful not to give electrolytes, e.g. potassium, too quickly for the patient and seek specialist advice if the patient is diabetic or blood glucose is raised following a step-up in rate. Typical longer-term, stable patients often end up receiving their IVN over 10–16 hours, usually overnight to permit more freedom during the day.

Recommencing intravenous nutrition after a period of inadequate feeding

Longer-term IVN patients, including those on home IVN, can be at risk from excessive IVN provision if, for any reason, there is a prolonged break in IVN administration. The most common reason for this is an episode of catheter-related sepsis when IVN is stopped in order to treat it (see Chapter 12). Recommencement of the IVN regimen may then need to be at a reduced rate, although it can often be increased fairly swiftly depending on clinical condition and tolerance. For a patient who has missed up to 5 days of IVN, you can usually restart at the full-rate that was previously prescribed (providing that the patient is now well and stable). If more than 5 days' treatment was missed or the patient remains unstable, a reduced initial rate is required. Reduced rates similar to those advocated above for shorter-term, sick patients should be used if a longer-term patient has had any significant intervention such as major surgery.

Specialised macronutrients

Most commercial IVN component manufacturers have a variety of macronutrient options from which to choose and keeping a range of products locally helps in designing your own regimens (see Chapter 11). The differences between the different brands' main products have traditionally been limited and hence, for example, a 14 gram nitrogen per litre product from two different companies would be interchangeable for most purposes except stability considerations. More recently, however, companies have started to adopt specialised products warranting particular consideration.

Specialised lipids

The theoretical disadvantages of the standard long-chain triglycerides (see above) have led to the development of several alternatives which vary in the fatty-acid chains attached to the glycerol backbone. However, it is neither possible nor desirable to exclude completely long-chain triglycerides since they include essential fatty acids and their slower metabolism can be useful. Newer classes of lipid products include the following:

- *Medium-chain triglycerides*: these are usually obtained from coconut oil[21] rather than soybean oil, which is the traditional source for IVN long-chain triglycerides. The fatty acids are 8–12 carbons in length compared to the longer 16–20 carbon chains of the traditional lipids. The shorter medium-chain triglycerides can be cleared from the blood stream more rapidly than long-chain triglycerides and this may improve tolerance and limit long-term adverse effects on the liver.
- *Structured medium-chain lipids*: these contain both long-chain and short-chain fatty acids on the same glycerol backbone rather than one or the other, as found in a physical mixture of long-chain and medium-chain fatty acids.
- *Olive oil-based*: these lipid products contain a high proportion of the monounsaturated fatty acid, oleic acid. This may reduce oxidative damage[22] and improve immune function, blood glucose

and lipid profiles in shorter-term patients. In longer-term IVN they may even offer Mediterranean-type diet benefits such as limiting atherosclerotic complications.

- *Fish oil-based*: these contain a much higher proportion of long-chain ω_3 fatty acids such as eicosapentaenoic acid and docosapentaenoic acid, relative to the n_6 series. The lipid may therefore reduce proinflammatory activity (see above).
- *Combination products*: Lipidem contains long-chain and medium-chain triglycerides as well as fish oil and SMOFlipid contains these plus olive oil. These products are intended to offer the advantages of each of the components that they contain.

Some of the commercially available range of lipids now available are shown in Table 7.9.

There have already been many studies comparing novel lipids to traditional long-chain triglyceride-containing IVN but interpretation is difficult for a number of reasons, including:

- Low subject numbers
- Overprovision of energy or different levels of energy given to one test group
- Unbalanced glucose-to-lipid ratios or excessive lipid provision
- Trials conducted in patients not typical of those supported by IVN

The advantages of the various novel lipids, therefore remain largely theoretical at present and the routine use of standard long-chain triglycerides[23] seems to be safe as long as they are prescribed sensibly with careful monitoring (see Chapter 13). However, there does seem to be a place for trying these novel products when patients show intolerance to traditional lipids (see Chapter 12), especially in patients on long-term IVN support. Further research will no doubt clarify their place in both short- and long-term IVN use.

Specialised nitrogen sources

Patients are likely to have abnormal AA demands during catabolism and the acute-phase response. This makes matching provision to actual needs difficult, as it is still unclear which AAs are needed and in what quantity. One possibility that is being investigated very actively at present is that high levels of glutamine provision grant advantage.

Catabolism leading to net protein loss is associated with a concurrent net loss in glutamine, which may then contribute to further protein loss[24]. Plasma levels of glutamine fall during illness but flux

Table 7.9 Examples of commercial lipids for use in intravenous nutrition formulation

Type of lipid emulsion*	Lipid name and manufacturer†	Comments
Long-chain triglyceride	Ivelip (Baxter), Lipofundin (B Braun), Intralipid (Fresenius Kabi)	This is the traditional lipid but is rapidly being overtaken by novel products as the standard lipid choice from manufacturers
Long-chain triglycerides with medium-chain triglycerides	Lipofundin S (B Braun), Structolipid (Fresenius Kabi)	B Braun uses a physical mixture of long-chain and medium-chain fatty acids which are on separate glycerol backbones, whereas Fresenius Kabi uses a chemical mixture so the fatty acids may or may not be on the same glycerol backbones
Olive oil (primarily) with long-chain triglycerides	Clinoleic (Baxter)	80% of the lipid is olive oil
Medium-chain triglycerides, long-chain triglycerides and fish oil	Lipidem (B Braun)	20% of the lipid is fish oil; the long-chain and medium-chain fatty acids are on separate triglycerides
Long-chain triglycerides, medium-chain triglycerides, olive oil and fish oil	SMOFLipid (Fresenius Kabi)	The medium-chain fatty acids are a physical mixture, not a chemical mixture as found in Structolipid (above)

* May have egg phospholipids or soybean phospholipids as an emulsifying agent and some may contain vitamin E.
† Companies listed in alphabetical order.

increases massively, so that glutamine supplies become huge. Nevertheless, demands may be greater still and hence additional supply may be helpful, although it would be expected that only very large quantities would make a significant difference. Specific supplementation of IVN using large doses of glutamine is suggested to offer benefits that include improved immune and antioxidative function, and reduced complications, length of stay and (late) mortality, depending on the patient population studied. However, large, well-designed studies are still required to prove this one way or the other[24].

Currently, the practice of using glutamine in IVN regimens is variable, as clear and consistent interpretation of the literature is often difficult (as with specialised lipids above). If you intend to use glutamine in an IVN regimen, always confirm stability with the manufacturer before prescribing.

References

1. Martin A. *Physical Pharmacy*, 4th edn. London: Lea and Febiger, 1993: 394.
2. Needle R, Sizer T, eds. *The CIVAS Handbook: The Centralised Intravenous Additive Services Reference*. London: Pharmaceutical Press, 1998: 67–68.
3. Kane K, Cologiovanni L, McKiernan *et al*. High osmolality feedings do not increase the incidence of thrombophlebitis during peripheral iv nutrition. *J Parenteral Enteral Nutr* 1996; 20: 194–197.
4. British Medical Association and the Royal Pharmaceutical Society of Great Britain. *British National Formulary* 36. London: British Medical Association and the Royal Pharmaceutical Society of Great Britain, 1998: 410.
5. Elia M. Insights into energy requirements in disease. Public Health Nutr 2005; 8: 1037–1052.
6. NICE and the National Collaborating Centre For Acute Care. *Nutrition Support in Adults: Oral Nutrition Support, Enteral Tube Feeding and Parenteral Nutrition*. London: NICE and the National Collaborating Centre For Acute Care, 2006.
7. Jeejeebhoy K. Rhoads lecture – 1988. Bulk or bounce – the object of nutritional support. *J Parenteral and Enteral Nutr* 1988; 12: 539–549.
8. van den Burghe G, Wouters P, Weekers F *et al*. Intensive insulin therapy in the critically ill patients. *N Engl J Med* 2001; 345: 1359–1367.
9. Krishnan J, Parce P, Martinez A *et al*. Caloric intake in medical ICU patients: consistency of care with guidelines and relationship to clinical outcomes. *Chest* 2003; 124: 297–305.
10. Carlson G. Insulin resistance and glucose-induced thermogenesis in critical illness. *Proc Nutr Soc* 2001; 60: 381–388.
11. Saeed M, Carlson G, Little R, Irving M. Selective impairment of glucose storage in human sepsis. *Br J Surg* 1999; 86: 813–821.
12. Buchman A. *Handbook of Nutritional Support*. Pennsylvania: Williams and Wilkins, 1997: 14.
13. Press M. Essential fatty acids (EFA). In: Karran S, Alberti K, eds. *Practical Nutritional Support*. London: Pitman Medical, 1980: 116–125.
14. Payne-James, Grimble G, Silk D, eds. *Artificial Nutrition Support in Clinical Practice*, 2nd edn. London: Greenwich Medical Media, 2001: 449.
15. Reeds P, Fjeld C, Jahoor F. Do the differences between the amino acid compositions of acute-phase and muscle proteins have a bearing on nitrogen loss in traumatic states? *J Nutr* 1994; 124: 906–910.
16. Klein C, Stanek G, Wiles C. Overfeeding macronutrients to critically ill adults: metabolic complications. *J Am Dietetic Assoc* 1998; 98: 795–806.
17. Peck M, Alexander J, Gonce S, Miskell P. Low protein diets improve survival from peritonitis in guinea pigs. *Ann Surg* 1989; 209: 448–454.

18. Collins S, Myatt M, Golden B. Dietary treatment of severe malnutrition in adults. *Am J Clin Nutr* 1998; 68: 193–199.
19. Scherbaum V, Furst P. New concepts on nutritional management of severe malnutrition: the role of protein. *Curr Opin Clin Nutr Metab Care* 2000; 3: 31–38.
20. Pennington C, ed. *Current Perspectives on Parenteral Nutrition in Adults.* Maidenhead: British Association for Parenteral and Enteral Nutrition, 1996: 13–14.
21. Fiaccadori E, Tortorella G, Gonzi G *et al*. Hemodynamic and respiratory effects of medium-chain and long-chain triglyceride fat emulsions: a prospective, randomized study. *Riv Ital Nutr Parenterale Enterale* 1997; 15: 6–14.
22. Payne-James J, Grimble G, Silk D, eds. *Artificial Nutrition Support in Clinical Practice*, 2nd edn. London: Greenwich Medical Media, 2001: 419.
23. Wanten G. An update on parenteral lipids and immune function: only smoke, or is there any fire? *Curr Opin Clin Nutr Metab Care* 2006: 9: 79–83.
24. Novak F, Heyland D, Avenell A *et al*. Glutamine supplementation in serious illness: a systematic review of the evidence. *Crit Care Med* 2002; 30: 2022–2029.

8

Electrolytes in intravenous nutrition

Introduction

The correct provision of electrolytes to intravenous nutrition (IVN) patients is arguably even more important than the correct levels of macronutrients and balance issues can be complex. Not only does IVN itself contain many different electrolytes in variable amounts but most IVN recipients receive many electrolytes from other intravenous fluids and drugs. Regulatory mechanisms may also be disturbed and both starvation and stress can in themselves alter electrolyte balance. This chapter aims to promote an understanding of the electrolyte requirements of IVN patients to ensure best prescribing and monitoring.

Balance and imbalance

A well-nourished individual operating normal homeostatic mechanisms is able to balance the input, output and distribution of body electrolytes (Figure 8.1).

The homeostatic mechanisms usually control electrolyte levels within tight limits but in the case of IVN patients, they are often deranged from:

- The effects of starvation and physiological stress
- Excessive losses of fluid and electrolytes
- Abnormalities in renal electrolyte handling
- Provision of electrolytes from multiple sources
- Drugs' effects on electrolyte regulation

Details of the effects of these different factors are given below.

Electrolytes, starvation and physiological stress

During starvation, patients consume relatively small amounts of electrolytes yet continue to excrete them (Figure 8.1). In addition, starvation

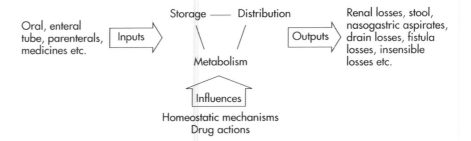

Figure 8.1 Electrolyte balance.

itself leads to the downregulation of many basal metabolic functions in order to save energy. This includes a reduction in the activity of the sodium–potassium and other membrane pumps, which usually maintain concentration gradients between intracellular and extracellular electrolyte levels. As a consequence, predominantly intracellular substances such as potassium, magnesium and phosphate leak out through cell membranes. They are then excreted by the kidney. This precipitates a state of total body intracellular electrolyte depletion in most starved patients, which is usually present even if reported serum levels are normal.

The starvation-related changes in membrane pumps also cause extracellular sodium and water to move into cells. Malnourished patients therefore tend to have high body salt and water content, which can be further exacerbated by iatrogenic salt and water administration (particularly since starvation also limits the kidneys' capacity to excrete a salt and water load). Furthermore, in many IVN patients there is elevation of circulating cortisol and aldosterone as a consequence of their physiological response to illness or injury. This also leads to sodium and water retention with simultaneous renal potassium loss. Great care is therefore needed to limit the provision of salt and water in most IVN patients while providing adequate potassium, magnesium and phosphate, and failure to do so can cause fluid overload, oedema and delayed resolution of gut dysfunction if it is due to ileus. It may also put them in danger of the life-threatening refeeding syndrome (see below).

Excessive losses of fluid and electrolytes

Since most patients requiring IVN have intestinal failure, the majority will also have abnormal fluid and electrolyte losses. The nature of these varies with the source and so it is essential not only to monitor the volume of fluid loss but also to consider its type and likely content. For example, gastric losses from vomiting or nasogastric drainage contain high levels of potassium and acid whereas small-bowel losses from drains, enterocutaneous fistulae or high ileal or jejunal stomas typically contain large quantities of sodium and magnesium, and may be very alkaline.

Abnormalities in renal electrolyte handling

In addition to intestinal failure, many IVN patients have varying degrees of renal impairment. In some, this is directly due to the dehydration from little or no oral or enteral fluid intake, perhaps coupled with the excessive salt and water losses from the gastrointestinal tract. In others, it is simply one of the many consequences of severe illness or injury since these are often accompanied by poor renal perfusion or a 'toxic' reduction in renal function. This is particularly true in patients with any pre-existing kidney disease such as diabetes. Whatever the cause, one of the main consequences of renal impairment is abnormal electrolyte handling and you must account for renal problems in your prescribing (see Chapter 10).

Provision of electrolytes from multiple sources

Most patients referred for IVN are receiving electrolytes from multiple sources and it is important to assess the total provision of each electrolyte, along with the patient's current biochemistry, renal function and likely losses, before deciding on their IVN prescription.

Different oral and enteral feeds contain variable concentrations of electrolytes per unit volume and so you will need to refer to manufacturers' information to evaluate any intakes from these routes. Similarly, you will need to account for the electrolyte content of some drugs, which can be very significant. Conversion between units from milligrams to millimoles is often needed (see Appendix 2). Intravenous antibiotics tend to be particularly high in sodium and Tazocin, for example, contains 9.4 mmol of sodium per 4.5-g vial[1]. This may not sound like much but, when administered three times daily in 100 ml 0.9% w/v sodium chloride, giving this drug alone contributes an additional 74.4 mmol sodium daily. Of course, intravenous fluids often contain electrolytes (see Chapter 7), either when manufactured or because of deliberate additions. The sodium provision from 0.9% w/v sodium chloride can be enormous since it contains 154 mmol/litre compared to normal requirements, which are typically only 1–2 mmol/kg per day (see below).

Drug effects on electrolyte regulation

Some drugs not only contain electrolytes but also have pharmacological effects on electrolyte balance. These side-effects are listed in the *British National Formulary* (BNF)[2], with the most common potential problems listed first. However, the BNF gives no information on the frequency of problems in practice and this information is only found in specialist sources such as the electronic Medicines Compendium[3], textbooks such as 'Meyler'[4] or 'Davies'[5] or directly from the medicine manufacturers. These sources may also tell you the mechanism of the effect which may guide your management. For example, furosemide causes increased renal excretion of potassium[6] whereas amphotericin causes increased renal excretion of potassium and magnesium[7]. The aim of treatment in any resulting hypokalaemia from these drugs should therefore be replacement rather than redistribution (Figure 8.1).

Interpreting biochemical results

Changes in electrolyte levels reported by chemical pathology are dependent on many factors, including total body content, tissue and fluid distribution and different sampling and analysis techniques. You therefore need to be cautious when interpreting analytical results since reported levels may have little relevance to whole-body status and prescribing needs.

Plasma electrolyte measurements

One of the most important factors to remember when interpreting plasma electrolyte values is whether the electrolyte is normally found predominantly intracellularly or extracellularly. Those found primarily within cells (e.g. potassium, magnesium and phosphate) are usually able to compensate for a drop in the plasma level by redistribution (Figure 8.2). In one sense this is useful since it reduces the level of change in the circulation but in another it can be misleading, since whole-body deficiency and intracellular depletion may affect function, yet not be reflected in reported biochemistry. However, when you do see a low reported serum level of a primarily intracellular electrolyte, there is

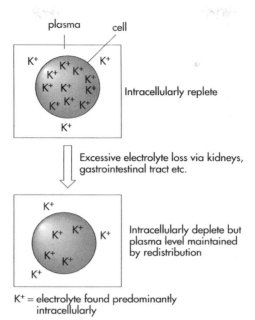

plasma   cell

Intracellularly replete

Excessive electrolyte loss via kidneys, gastrointestinal tract etc.

Intracellularly deplete but plasma level maintained by redistribution

K⁺ = electrolyte found predominantly intracellularly

Figure 8.2 Reported biochemistry does not necessarily reflect the total body level of primarily intracellular electrolytes.

Notes: Reported biochemistry shows a low level at stage (K). Careful interpretation of any reported biochemistry is always important.

almost certainly significant total body depletion since intracellular contents can no longer be high enough to replenish the plasma.

For predominantly extracellular electrolytes such as sodium the laboratory reported plasma levels may reflect total body content but in practice they rarely do so. The reason for this is that the reported extracellular concentrations are dramatically affected by fluid balance (Figure 8.3). Low serum sodiums, often seen in sick IVN-type patients, are most commonly due to excessive total body water rather than whole-body sodium depletion and, indeed, total sodium in such patients is often high. The best treatment for hyponatraemia in most IVN patients is therefore more likely to be reduced fluid administration with monitoring of renal function and urine output, rather than increased sodium provision, which may make salt and water retention worse. Measurement of urinary electrolytes can be helpful in determining the best course of action (see below).

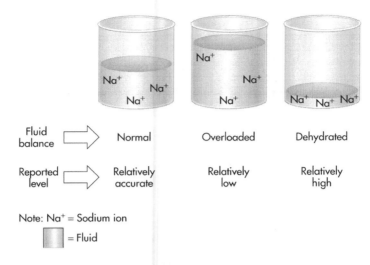

Figure 8.3 How fluid balance can affect reported sodium biochemistry.

Urinary electrolyte measurements

Electrolytes are charged (Appendix 2), water-soluble and, in most cases, primarily excreted and regulated by the kidney. If your patient has total body depletion of an electrolyte, the kidneys are therefore likely to try to maintain levels by reducing urinary loss (Figure 8.1). Measurement of urinary electrolytes is therefore a valuable tool in determining whole-body status and likely IVN prescribing needs, as long as the kidneys are themselves working properly.

A single sodium measurement on a random urinary sample is usually adequate to help in determining true body sodium status in patients with abnormal plasma levels and fluid imbalance. A low result of < 50 mmol/L and especially < 25 mmol/L strongly suggests total body sodium depletion and hence that more sodium should be administered. Conversely, a level of > 150 mmol/L suggests that your patient is receiving too much sodium and/or is trying to excrete a previous excess sodium load. Less must therefore be prescribed. Although 24-hour urinary collections are more accurate, they involve more work and are not usually required.

Interpretation of urinary electrolytes can be problematic, however, if the patient:

- Has renal impairment, which can cause abnormal retention or losses

- Has neuroendocrine changes that cause abnormal electrolyte handling (e.g. raised cortisol in physiological stress, exogenous administration of steroids; raised aldosterone in physiological stress, low blood pressure, dehydration, liver disease or raised antidiuretic hormone, which is usually caused by drugs, chest infections or with some tumours)
- Is on drugs that influence renal electrolyte handling, such as diuretics that can force electrolyte loss

Abnormal status of one electrolyte can also lead to abnormal renal handling of another. Renal potassium retention, for example, is usually accompanied by increased sodium loss, whereas magnesium depletion promotes renal potassium loss. In the case of calcium and magnesium, both plasma and urinary levels are difficult to interpret because of the potential release from the stores within the skeleton.

Electrolyte monitoring

In order to identify and correct any problems in electrolyte balance, you need to monitor electrolyte levels in plasma (and sometimes urine) regularly, bearing in mind the limitations of the plasma measurements, as discussed above. Reported plasma levels are compared to reference ranges rather than reference values since there is a natural variation in electrolyte levels, even within the same patient. The ranges used are based on measurements in healthy populations and are validated using specific testing methods. However, different analytical methods result in different measurements for the same electrolyte and so local reference ranges are not interchangeable. All patients on IVN need initial careful electrolyte monitoring on a daily basis. Details are given in Chapter 13. Additional clinical monitoring, e.g. using an electrocardiogram, may be indicated when serum electrolytes are very abnormal.

Before prescribing IVN, you should ideally examine several days of previous biochemistry to look for trends to guide you. A recent rise or fall in reported electrolyte levels can be a useful indicator of the onset or resolution of renal compromise, excessive or inadequate electrolyte provision and changes in levels of loss. Inconsistent or very acute changes in biochemistry suggest that they may be spurious and need rechecking. Common causes of spurious abnormalities include:

- Contamination of the sample from IVN or other intravenous fluid administered distally into the sample vein
- Haemolysis of the sample prior to measurement of the electrolyte

levels. This causes release of the intracellular contents of blood cells and consequently artificially high levels of potassium, magnesium and phosphate (note that a sample showing hyperkalaemia without confirmation of haemolysis may still have been haemolysed and it is important to check with the laboratory that haemolysis was not present)

If any problems are suspected, urgent rechecking of biochemistry may be needed and it must be remembered that evidence of haemolysis does not exclude the possibility that there is also a problem of genuinely high levels of one or more serum electrolytes.

Consequences of electrolyte imbalance

Although plasma electrolyte levels do not necessarily reflect total body status, they are critically important in maintaining organ function. Some tolerance to levels outside the normal ranges is possible, especially if the onset of the abnormality is slow. However, levels that are either very high or very low, and changes in either direction that have occurred quickly, pose considerable dangers. Some of the most serious consequences of abnormal serum electrolyte levels are shown in Table 8.1.

Reintroduction of feeding by any route in a malnourished patient can lead to very rapid onset of severe electrolyte abnormalities, including hypokalaemia, hypomagnesaemia and hypophosphataemia. These are often coupled with sodium and fluid retention and vitamin abnormalities, with the whole problem known as the refeeding syndrome.

The refeeding syndrome

The refeeding syndrome occurs as a result of reintroduction of nutrition after a period of inadequate nutritional intake. The effects may be profound and can put the patient at grave risk. They occur with the reintroduction of nutrition by any route but are more common with enteral tube feeding and IVN[8,9]. The classical refeeding syndrome is mainly related to abnormalities of electrolyte and fluid balance but the use of nutrition support without adequate micronutrients also results in other refeeding complications, such as the Wernicke–Korsakoff syndrome (see Chapter 9).

As discussed above, sodium is primarily found extracellularly whereas potassium, magnesium and phosphate are primarily intracellular. This is due to active pumping mechanisms, including the

Table 8.1 Common potential consequences of abnormal serum electrolytes

Electrolyte	Low	High
Sodium	Nausea, vomiting, headache, hypotension, malaise, stupor, coma	Muscle weakness, confusion, hypertension
Potassium	Muscle weakness, hypotonia, depression, paralytic ileus, confusion, arrhythmias	Electrocardiogram changes, malaise, palpitations, muscle weakness
Magnesium	Irritability, tremor, confusion, convulsions, electrocardiogram changes	Weakness, respiratory paralysis, defects in cardiac conduction
Calcium	Paraesthesia, tetany	Fatigue, confusion, nausea, vomiting, abdominal pain, higher urine output, abnormal heart rhythms, (renal or bladder stones if chronic)
Phosphate	Muscle weakness, muscle wasting, skeletal wasting	Chronic renal failure, hypoparathyroidism

sodium–potassium pump. During a prolonged period of inadequate nutrition the body attempts to compensate for the lack of nutrient intake by reducing all energy-consuming metabolic processes. As part of this downregulation, the activity of cellular pumps is reduced, causing electrolytes to leak across cell membranes. This leads to potassium, magnesium and phosphate moving into the plasma followed by their renal excretion and the development of total body deficits. Simultaneously, sodium leaks into the cells, a change which is accompanied by an increase in intracellular water content.

The introduction of nutrition by any route results in a reactivation of cellular pumping mechanisms along with a carbohydrate-induced release of insulin to move glucose into cells. These processes cause a sudden increase in the movement of potassium, magnesium and phosphate from plasma to cell interiors while simultaneously there is a rapid movement of sodium and water from within the cells into the circulation. The sodium–potassium pump also utilises magnesium as a cofactor[10], which further reduces magnesium availability, and the deficit of phosphate is worsened by the sudden increase in the intracellular manufacture of energy-storing adenosine triphosphate. The net result of these processes can be acute hypokalaemia, hypomagnesaemia and hypophosphataemia, often coupled with rapid circulatory overload from sodium and water moving out of the cells, especially as malnutrition limits the renal capacity to excrete a salt and water load. Furthermore, the introduction of nutrition is often accompanied by the administration of further intravenous fluids and the potential for iatrogenic salt and water overload. Patients may therefore suffer from a wide variety of problems, including acute cardiac failure, cardiac arrhythmias and sudden death. Neurological complications such as convulsions or coma can also occur.

Risks of refeeding syndrome

All patients who have had very little nutritional intake for more than 5 days (i.e. most referrals for IVN) are at some risk of refeeding problems. Nutrition support should therefore be commenced at a maximum of 50% of requirements for 2 days in most patients. Full needs can then be met later if clinical and biochemical monitoring reveals no refeeding problems. Even greater care is needed in some patients, particularly those meeting any one of the following criteria:

- Body mass index (BMI) < 16 kg/m^2
- Unintentional weight loss of > 15% within the previous 3–6 months
- Very little or no nutrient intake for > 10 days
- Low levels of potassium, phosphate or magnesium prior to any feeding.

Patients with two or more of the following lesser criteria are also at high refeeding risk:

- BMI < 18.5 kg/m^2
- Unintentional weight loss > 10% within the previous 3–6 months
- Very little or no intake for > 5 days
- A history of alcohol abuse or some drugs, including insulin, chemotherapy, antacids or diuretics.

Individual electrolyte considerations

Sodium

Sodium is primarily found in the extracellular compartment and is uniquely influenced by total body water levels (Figure 8.3). Excessive fluid and dehydration therefore result in difficulties in interpreting reported sodium levels (Table 8.2), although urinary measures may help (see above).

Table 8.2 Potential complication of fluid on interpreting reported sodium levels in your patient's biochemistry*

Serum sodium →	Low	Normal	High
Fluid status ↓			
Dehydrated	Normonatraemia, hypernatraemia	Hypernatraemia	Hypernatraemia
Normal fluid balance	Hyponatraemia	Normonatraemia	Hypernatraemia
Fluid-overloaded	Hyponatraemia	Hyponatraemia	Normonatraemia, hyponatraemia

* Always consider whether other mechanisms may be affecting sodium status, including hormonal and drug effects. Hyponatraemia may be also be caused by a genuine total body sodium deficit, just as hypernatraemia may be caused by a genuine total body excess.

Excessive provision of sodium and fluid is a particularly common problem in IVN patients. The problem is usually caused by too much normal saline being given to patients either before the IVN referral, particularly in those who are postoperative, or after IVN has been started because the non-nutrition team prescribers forget to account for the sodium and fluid content of the IVN regimen. These problems not only result in oedema and, in some cases, in breathlessness from left ventricular failure, but can also cause persistence in the ileus which often underlies the IVN referral. Greater care, with reduced postoperative saline administration, has been shown to grant considerable advantage. Studies in patients having elective colonic resection, for example, show that sodium and fluid administration sufficient to cause a 3-kg weight gain delays recovery of gut function and prolongs hospital stay. Furthermore, if patients are relatively saline-restricted they have fewer complications, heal better and have higher levels of serum albumin[11,12].

Inadequate provision of sodium is less common than saline overload but genuine sodium depletion can occur in IVN patients with excess losses e.g. from high-output stomas or caused by diuretics. Dilutional hyponatraemia from excessive administration of intravenous glucose also occurs and low sodiums are seen in patients with the syndrome of inappropriate antidiuretic hormone (SIADH) who have dilution of all plasma components. This occurs most frequently in patients with chest infections, some malignancies and with some drugs.

Hyponatraemia causes the symptoms shown in Table 8.1, especially if the onset is rapid. Of even more concern is overrapid correction, especially if low levels have been present for some days. This can lead to pontine demyelination and even death and hence very cautious correction is indicated (more rapid correction can be used if the fall in serum sodium has been acute and short-lived but nevertheless is probably best avoided).

Likely prescribing needs

The standard provision of sodium in IVN is 40–70 mmol/day (Box 8.1) but it is not usually necessary to worry if you are providing less than this (e.g. when starting regimens at half-rate; see Chapter 7). This is because supplemental intravenous fluids or drugs are usually providing considerable additional sodium. However, if the patient's sole source of sodium is the IVN and there is no clinical indication to restrict sodium input, you may need to adjust the low levels of sodium found in some standard commercial IVN bags (30–40 mmol) to meet the normal daily needs (around 60–70 mmol). Extra sodium is also needed in patients with very high sodium losses, particularly those with high-output fistulae or stomas, who can lose hundreds of millimoles per day (see Chapter 10). If necessary, check the stability of large sodium additions before prescribing.

Patients who are fluid- and sodium-overloaded, including those with liver disease and ascites, will almost certainly require restriction on

---

Box 8.1 Providing or adjusting sodium in intravenous nutrition (IVN) regimens

Typical daily requirement
40–70 mmol or 0.8 mmol/kg

Typical variations
Short-bowel syndrome – likely need may be hundreds of millimoles per day (see Chapter 10)

Oedema or ascites – 30–50 mmol or even less (0–30 mmol) if receiving sodium from other sources, e.g. intravenous drugs (see Chapter 5)

Typical clinical significance of adjustments
Usually in multiples of 40 mmol unless there is short-bowel syndrome, when adjustments of 50–100 mmol are more appropriate

±10–20 mmol from that intended to prescribe is unlikely to be clinically significant unless the IVN is the only sodium source

Note: always review requirements in the context of patient assessment (see Chapter 4) and the stability of the proposed regimen (see Appendix 1)

the sodium content of their IVN, often with a concurrent volume restriction. This usually applies even when their serum sodium is low, since the hyponatraemia is usually the result of sodium retention (with high total body content) coupled with an even greater level of water retention (see Chapter 10).

Potassium

Potassium is primarily found intracellularly. Wards often refer to administration of grams of potassium chloride, so conversion between mmol and grams is frequently needed (Equation 8.1).

1 g potassium chloride = 13.5 mmol potassium
(approximate conversion)   (Eqn 8.1)

As discussed above, the primarily intracellular location of potassium means that reported plasma levels may not reflect total body levels and although a reported hypokalaemic value will usually indicate total body potassium depletion, individuals with considerable whole-body depletion may still have normal plasma levels.

High plasma potassiums may be due to genuine total body excess, increased *in vivo* release of potassium from within cells (e.g. that seen with extensive cell damage from haemolysis, injury or sepsis), or reduced potassium excretion due to renal impairment. It can also be an *ex vivo* artefact from haemolysis during or following venesection.

Low plasma potassiums are usually seen in patients with high losses (e.g. with diarrhoea), those with an inadequate intake and those suffering from the refeeding syndrome (see above). Excess renal potassium losses can occur even when total body levels are low as the renal system may be unable to retain potassium effectively, e.g. with magnesium deficiency[13] or potassium-losing drugs, including some diuretics.

Likely prescribing needs

The standard potassium IVN provision is 60 mmol/day, usefully altered in multiples of 20 mmol subject to stability constraints (Box 8.2). Excessive potassium losses will need replacing and significant diarrhoea or vomiting, for example, result in increased requirements[14] e.g. up to 2–3 times normal and occasionally even more. Patients with renal compromise can have difficulty with urinary excretion of potassium and very low levels in the IVN may be needed to prevent dangerous plasma accumulation (0–20 mmol/day).

Box 8.2 Providing or adjusting potassium in intravenous nutrition regimens

Typical daily requirement
60 mmol or 0.9 mmol/kg

Higher standard provision during the initial stages of refeeding if at high risk of refeeding complications (see text)

Prescribing on a mmol/kg basis preferred for low-weight patients

Typical variations
High losses, e.g. severe diarrhoea or high nasogastric tube output, can require hundreds of millimoles but increase with care

Electrolyte-retaining renal impairment: 0–20 mmol per day

Typical clinical significance of adjustments
Usually in multiples of 20 mmol: 1 multiple is a definite change, 2 a large change and 3 or more multiples a very large change

±5–10 mmol is unlikely to be clinically significant providing there is still some prescribed and the patient has a standard requirement

Note: always review requirements in the context of patient assessment (see Chapter 4) and the stability of the proposed regimen (see Appendix 1)

IVN patients may be receiving potassium supplementation from sources additional to their IVN, e.g. potassium chloride in intravenous infusions. It is often possible to reduce or even eliminate the requirement for these by adding more potassium to the IVN regimen. This can simplify matters for the ward staff and may help to limit unwanted additional fluids being given to the patient. However, the addition of extra potassium to IVN should only be undertaken when you have identified the reason for the higher potassium requirement and understand how this may change over time. Clear communication with all ward and other medical staff involved is essential, in order to ensure that patients do not receive additional potassium in their IVN as well as extra potassium from other infusions. You must also account for any decline in the patient's requirement for potassium when prescribing further IVN, e.g. with resolution of diarrhoea or nasogastric tube losses. A review of existing IVN that is running may be needed in some circumstances.

Interactions can occur between potassium regulation and the regulation of other electrolytes, and these may influence prescribing needs. It is very difficult for the body to excrete an excess sodium and water load when there is a potassium shortage for exchange in the kidney. Generous potassium provision should therefore be given to oedematous patients, with plasma levels run at the upper end of the normal range. Similarly, as noted above, hypokalaemia is almost impossible to correct in the face of magnesium deficiency with high renal potassium loss. Persistent hypokalemia may therefore require high levels of magnesium provision as well as generous potassium prescribing[15].

IVN patients who have previously been very undernourished are likely to be depleted in whole-body potassium, magnesium and phosphate (see above). This patient group might therefore also benefit from maintaining plasma levels at the upper end of the normal range since this should maximise correction rates of the low levels within cells while minimising risks of the precipitous drops in levels that can occur with refeeding. Clinicians may also aim to run relatively high potassium levels in some cardiac patients with arrhythmic risk (see Chapter 10).

Magnesium

Magnesium is primarily found intracellularly. It may not be routinely reported with urea and electrolytes requests and must therefore be specifically requested. High levels are seen most frequently in renal impairment, iatrogenic administration and with sample haemolysis. Low levels may not reflect true total body status but genuine magnesium depletion is seen in patients with excessive diarrhoea or high stomal losses, and with starvation as part of the refeeding syndrome (see above).

Likely prescribing needs

The standard provision of magnesium in IVN is 5 mmol/day, usefully altered in increments of a further 5 mmol subject to stability constraints (Box 8.3). However, compared to the standard, non-IVN, intravenous replacement of 5 g magnesium sulphate (approximately 20 mmol magnesium), the range of possible adjustment in IVN is limited (by stability – see Appendix 1). A very low plasma magnesium may therefore require additional, separate intravenous infusion of magnesium, taking care to avoid administration through the same lumen as the IVN in order to avoid precipitation risks. The addition of further magnesium in the IVN should not stop the administration of alternatively prescribed magnesium replacement and, conversely, additional prescribed magnesium should not stop increased provision in the IVN to help limit further depletion and the need for other supplementary sources. Patients

---

Box 8.3 Providing or adjusting magnesium in intravenous nutrition regimens

Typical daily requirement
5 mmol or 0.13 mmol/kg

Higher standard provision during the initial stages of refeeding if at high risk of refeeding complications (see text)

Typical variations
High losses, e.g. severe diarrhoea or high nasogastric tube output, can require up to about 15 mmol or even more subject to stability

Electrolyte-retaining renal impairment: 0–2.5 mmol per day

Typical clinical significance of adjustments
Usually in multiples of 5–10 mmol

±0–5 mmol is unlikely to be clinically significant provided there is still some prescribed and the patient has a standard requirement

Note: always review requirements in the context of patient assessment (see Chapter 4) and the stability of the proposed regimen (see Appendix 1)

---

with significant renal impairment will have difficulty excreting magnesium and very low levels may be needed in the IVN (0–2.5 mmol/day).

Calcium

Calcium is primarily found in the skeleton, where there are huge reserves. The plasma level does not therefore reflect whole-body status. Extracellular serum calcium is mainly present in two forms – either bound to albumin or as free ionised (or charged: see Appendix 2) calcium. It is the free, ionised form that is biologically active[16]. The reported laboratory values reflect both forms of calcium and so when serum albumin is high, the active proportion is relatively lower than that reported. Conversely, if the serum albumin level is low, the active proportion of the reported calcium is relatively higher than would be anticipated (Figure 8.4).

In view of the above, reported calcium levels are usually corrected for the patient's albumin level according to Equations 8.2–8.4[14,17], depending on the units used.

If serum albumin < 40 g/L, corrected calcium in mmol/L
= (serum calcium in mmol/L) + 0.02 (40 – (serum albumin in g/L))

(Eqn 8.2)

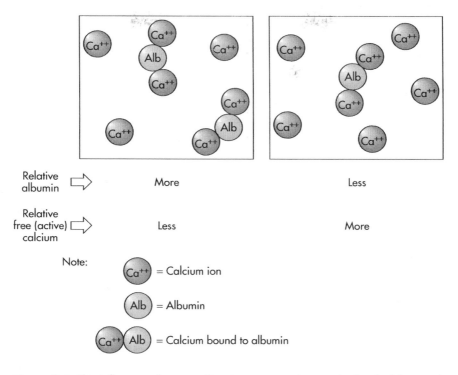

Note:

Ca^{++} = Calcium ion

Alb = Albumin

Ca^{++}Alb = Calcium bound to albumin

Figure 8.4 The influence of serum albumin concentration on the level of free and therefore active calcium.

If serum albumin > 45 g/L, corrected calcium in mmol/L
= (serum calcium in mmol/L) – 0.02 ((serum
albumin in g/L) – 45)   (Eqn 8.3)

Corrected calcium in mg/dL for a low serum calcium
= (serum calcium in mg/dL) + 0.8(4 – (serum
albumin in g/dL))   (Eqn 8.4)

All these calcium correction equations are inaccurate with very low plasma albumin levels. If plasma albumin is very low and the corrected figure is low but stable or increasing, replacement in addition to standard IVN quantities is not needed unless the patient is symptomatic (e.g. tetanic reaction). If the serum albumin is very low and the corrected calcium is low and falling, additional replacement is required.

A more accurate method of determining active calcium levels is to run a blood gas sample which reports only ionised calcium levels. If there is doubt over whether to replace calcium in the presence of a low albumin, this offers a quick method of determining best action. Blood gas reference ranges for calcium differ from laboratory reference ranges since they only measure ionised levels.

High calcium levels are primarily seen with hyperparathyroidism and renal failure but also occur in other conditions, including dehydration, hyperthyroidism, bone metastases, multiple myeloma and drug therapy (e.g. thiazide diuretics). Hypercalcaemia may also result from excessive calcium supplementation. Potential causes of low calcium levels are hypoparathyroidism, hypomagnaesaemia, hyperphosphataemia, drug therapy (e.g. furosemide) and deficiency of vitamin D, which is often due to a combination of inadequate dietary intake, poor absorption and a lack of exposure to sunlight. Low vitamin D activity is also seen in patients with either chronic kidney or liver disease, since the two hydroxylation steps needed for activation occur in these organs.

Bone is in a constant process of breakdown and deposition, with the balance of the two processes determining whether there is net loss or gain of bone density. Anything affecting this process may influence serum calcium levels and bisphosphonates, for example, may cause a fall in levels due to reduced bone breakdown.

Likely prescribing needs

Standard calcium IVN provision is 5 mmol/day and may be usefully altered in increments of 2.5 mmol subject to stability constraints (Box 8.4). A 2.5-mmol increment is a very similar quantity to standard intravenous calcium supplementation of 10 ml 10% w/v calcium gluconate (approximately 2.25 mmol calcium) and so addition of extra calcium to the IVN can often be used to avoid additional calcium needs unless supplementation is urgent. Sometimes large intravenous infusions of calcium are given (40 ml of 10% w/v calcium gluconate; about 10 mmol).

Care is needed when prescribing calcium and phosphate in IVN since they readily interact to form an insoluble precipitate (the same interaction that prevents concurrent oral or enteral tube administration of calcium and phosphate in order to avoid binding and subsequent non-absorption). You must also avoid the intravenous administration of either through the same lumen of an intravenous catheter as the IVN, since precipitatation can block the line or lead to pulmonary embolus.

Metastatic calcification is the deposition of calcium phosphate precipitate outside the skeletal system. It may result from a raised circulating concentration of calcium or phosphate[18] and excessive

Box 8.4 Providing or adjusting calcium in intravenous nutrition regimens

Typical daily requirement
5 mmol or 0.13 mmol/kg

Typical variations
Relatively uncommon

Typical clinical significance of adjustments
Usually in multiples of 2.5–5 mmol

±0–2.5 mmol is unlikely to be clinically significant, providing there is still some prescribed and the patient has a standard requirement

Note: always review requirements in the context of patient assessment (see Chapter 4) and the stability of the proposed regimen (see Appendix 1)

administration of either calcium or phosphate in the presence of high plasma levels of the other should always be avoided. For similar reasons, an increase in plasma calcium or phosphate may cause the other to drop and so excessive administration of either should be avoided if the plasma level of the other is low.

Phosphate

Phosphate is a primarily intracellular electrolyte but is also found in large quantities in the skeleton, where it is associated with calcium. Once again, therefore, reported plasma serum values do not reflect total body phosphate. Awareness of phosphate levels is an important part of nutritional assessment but they are often not reported routinely with urea and electrolytes requests. They should therefore be specifically asked for.

Hyperphosphataemia can result from sample haemolysis, renal compromise or excessive supplementation. Hypophosphataemia is usually due to total body depletion and is particularly common as part of the refeeding syndrome (see above).

Likely prescribing needs

Standard daily phosphate provision in IVN is 20–35 mmol and may usefully be altered in increments of 10–15 mmol subject to stability constraints (Box 8.5). Adjusting phosphate in an IVN regimen is

---

Box 8.5 Providing or adjusting phosphate in intravenous nutrition regimens

---

Typical daily requirement
20–35 mmol or 0.3–0.5 mmol/kg

Higher standard provision during the initial stages of refeeding if at high risk of refeeding complications (see text)

Typical variations
Electrolyte-retaining renal impairment: 0–5 mmol per day

Typical clinical significance of adjustments
Usually in multiples of 10 mmol

±0–5 mmol is unlikely to be clinically significant, providing there is still some prescribed and the patient has a standard requirement

Note: always review requirements in the context of patient assessment (see Chapter 4) and the stability of the proposed regimen (see Appendix 1)

---

therefore more likely to have a significant clinical effect than a standard, separate intravenous phosphate infusion of 10 mmol (see below).

Patients with renal impairment may have difficulty excreting phosphate and very low levels of provision may be needed (0–5 mmol/day). However, beware of the dehydrated, starving patient with prerenal kidney impairment and a consequent high phosphate. The administration of nutrients and fluids can rapidly restore renal phosphate clearance in such cases, while simultaneously the arrival of nutrients stimulates cellular phosphate uptake (part of the refeeding syndrome). The consequent change from very high to very low plasma phosphates can therefore be both dramatic and dangerous.

Lipid products within IVN always provide some phosphate in the form of phospholipids (see Chapter 7). The quantity provided within the lipid is usually very low (5 mmol or less of phosphate) and there is debate as to whether it should be included in the nominal IVN content since it is integral to the phospholipids and may not be readily available for cellular uptake. This book refers to total IVN phosphate rather than non-lipid phosphate.

Adequate phosphate should be provided to allow phosphorylation of glucose and the *BNF* suggests 20–30 mmol/day[19]. A patient who appears stable on lower levels of provision may in reality require more for optimal utilisation of glucose, particularly during initial stages of refeeding.

Standard electrolyte prescribing

Prescribing electrolytes in IVN for a 24-hour period may be based on:

- Standard total quantities of each electrolyte
- A standard mmol/kg of each electrolyte
- A combination of these approaches

Whichever method you use, you may well need to modify resulting values based on your individual patient.

Standard values for provision of electrolytes in IVN are shown in Table 8.3. For low-weight patients (40 kg or below), it may be more accurate to base initial electrolyte requirements on a mmol/kg basis rather than using the nominal values. Oedematous or obese patients will have a lower relative proportion of metabolically active cells and consideration should be given to initially using their ideal body weight instead of their actual body weight.

You will see in Chapter 15 that unnecessary electrolyte additions to IVN regimens create much more work for Technical Services (who compound the prescription) than might first be imagined. For this reason, you must ensure that any change you make to the electrolyte

Table 8.3 Summary of standard intravenous nutrition prescription electrolyte requirements*

Electrolyte	Nominal total mmol per 24-hour period	mmol/kg per 24-hour period	Notes
Sodium	40–70	0.8	60–70 mmol/day if no additional 0.9% w/v sodium chloride. Total per 24 hours 1–2 mmol/kg. Patients with short-bowel syndrome may have a much higher requirement
Potassium	60	0.9	
Magnesium	5	0.13	
Calcium	5	0.13	
Phosphate	20–35	0.3–0.5	The addition of phosphate may also unavoidably provide sodium, potassium or both (see Appendix 2)

* Subject to patient review and IVN regimen stability.

content of an IVN regimen is clinically relevant. For example, changing the potassium content by 2 mmol/day (from 60 to 62 or 58 mmol) is not likely to make any clinical difference but will waste time and resources.

Rates of administration

You should initially prescribe IVN to be administered as a continuous infusion in order to ensure consistency. If the first bag or two (depending on the rate; see Chapter 7) is to be administered over more than 24 hours, the electrolyte provision in each 24-hour period must be appropriate as far as regimen stability allows (see Appendix 1). In the case of a 48-hour bag, the required potassium, magnesium, calcium and phosphate per 24 hours will normally need to be doubled subject to stability constraints. However, it is not normally necessary to double the sodium content, especially as additional sodium provision from other sources is very likely if less than full-rate IVN is being given. Any additional fluid and electrolytes will usually be prescribed by the ward clinicians (see Chapter 4).

If the bag is run over less than 24 hours the patient may receive the whole bag contents or only a proportion of them depending on the prescribed rate. Always consider the electrolyte provision from the IVN per 24-hour period.

Change slowly and monitor

Where applicable, gradual changes in the IVN content are most appropriate with adequate monitoring (see Chapter 13). Remember that any regimen change that you make will not realistically be reflected for 24–48 hours after the infusion commences and that, if your newly prescribed regimen is started in the evening, the biochemistry from the following morning will not reflect the full effects of the change since the patient will have only received part of the altered regimen. In view of this, it is best to limit changes to prescribed regimens as far as possible, especially as this practice also improves the chances of being able to redirect an unused bag that has already been compounded.

In some cases more generous alterations to the IVN content are required, for example a patient with a very significant potassium requirement due to severe diarrhoea, vomiting or drug-induced losses.

Account for deficits

You will need to account for any electrolyte deficits of your patient as a result of excessive losses, but in the initial days of refeeding it is also necessary to account for masked deficits when appropriate. This will depend on the patient's nutritional history (see Chapter 4) but generally you should allow for the standard electrolyte provision per 24-hour period (above), even if the bag is run over more than 24 hours.

Intravenous nutrition stability

Your prescribing may be limited by the stability of the IVN regimen that you are prescribing so that it may not be possible to add the desired quantity of any electrolyte to any particular IVN regimen. Always prescribe within stability limits to limit the potential for significant complications such as pulmonary embolus from precipitation or regimen 'cracking', as well as inappropriate electrolyte provision (see Appendix 1).

Prescribing with risk of refeeding syndrome

Any patient at high risk of refeeding syndrome should commence feeding at very low levels of energy and protein provision with generous delivery of potassium, magnesium and phosphate, unless blood levels are already high (this may be the case if the patient also has renal impairment). High-dose thiamine and other B-group vitamins will also be needed to prevent other refeeding issues, such as Wernicke–Korsakoff syndrome, and balanced, generous multivitamin and trace element supplementation should be provided for all since the patients are likely to have multiple deficits that will not be met by low-level oral, enteral or intravenous feeding (see Chapter 9). Levels of feeding can then be increased over a few days if careful monitoring reveals no problems. The National Institute for Health and Clinical Excellence (NICE) recommendations for prescribing nutrition support in patients at high risk of refeeding problems are shown in Box 8.6.

It is important to appreciate that patients with normal prefeeding levels of potassium, magnesium and phosphate can still be at high risk of refeeding syndrome since many of those with high plasma levels will still have whole-body depletion. They are therefore still likely to need specific supplementation as refeeding progresses and renal function improves. Some authorities recommend prefeeding correction of any

Box 8.6 National Institute for Health and Clinical Excellence (NICE) recommendations on nutrition support in patients at high risk of refeeding problems[20]

- Start nutrition support at a maximum of 10 kcal/kg per day, increasing levels slowly to meet or exceed full needs by 4–7 days
- Use only 5 kcal/kg per day in extreme cases (e.g. body mass index < 14 kg/m² or negligible intake for more than 15 days) and monitor cardiac rhythm continually in these patients and others who either have or develop cardiac arrythmias
- Restore circulatory volume and monitor fluid balance and overall clinical status closely
- Provide immediately before and during the first 10 days of feeding: oral thiamine 200–300 mg daily, vitamin B compound strong 1 or 2 tablets three times a day (or full-dose daily intravenous vitamin B preparation, if necessary) and balanced multivitamin and trace element supplementation
- Provide oral, enteral or intravenous supplements of potassium (likely requirement 2–4 mmol/kg per day), phosphate (likely requirement 0.3–0.6 mmol/kg per day) and magnesium (likely requirement 0.2 mmol/kg per day intravenously or 0.4 mmol/kg per day oral/enteral) unless prefeeding plasma levels are high. Prefeeding correction of low plasma levels is unnecessary

existing electrolyte abnormalities, but this may provide a false sense of security. Total intracellular electrolyte deficits in severely malnourished patients can amount to hundreds of millimoles and little change in the deficit will occur unless supplementation is given with energy and other nutrients to encourage transmembrane transfer. High-risk patients therefore need electrolyte supplements with *simultaneous* commencement of feeding at *very low levels*. However, the IVN regimen may not supply enough of any specific electrolyte to correct any marked abnormality and hence specific supplementation may also be needed.

Correcting severe specific electrolyte abnormalities

Intravenous replacement of specific electrolytes is sometimes indicated either before commencement of IVN (when plasma levels are dangerously low) or with very cautious introduction of low-level feeding to promote cellular uptake. Do not plan on using IVN electrolyte additions for urgent replacement because IVN does not allow for rapid administration and the infusion may not begin for several hours after prescribing due to the time taken to compound the bag in Technical Services (see

Table 8.4 Typical intravenous electrolyte replacement to be modified according to local policy and patient's clinical condition*†

Electrolyte	Administration	Notes
Potassium	Usual maximum concentration of 40 mmol/litre and rate of 10 mmol/hour for peripheral administration. More concentrated or rapid infusion needs specialist facilities, including electrocardiogram monitoring. Very significant replacement would be 1 g to 2 g potassium chloride in 100 ml (or even 50 ml) over 1 hour administered centrally, subject to local policy and restrictions. Regular blood gas results are recommended for significant replacement	Use commercial premixed bags wherever possible; avoid rapid infusion unless necessary. 1 g potassium chloride is equivalent to approximately 13.5 mmol potassium
Magnesium	5 g magnesium sulphate in 50 mL 0.9% w/v sodium chloride given over 5 hours	Equivalent to approximately 20 mmol magnesium. May be given peripherally depending on veins. More limited replacement of 2 or 3 g magnesium sulphate may be more appropriate in some cases which can be given in 20 ml over 2 hours or 30 ml over 3 hours respectively
Calcium	10 mL of 10% w/v calcium gluconate given as a bolus or as an infusion in 50–100 mL of 0.9% w/v sodium chloride (over 30 minutes to 4 hours)	Equivalent to approximately 2.25 mmol calcium. Higher doses for infusion may be required in some cases. Give infusion over up to 24 hours but typically over 4 hours. May be given peripherally depending on veins
Phosphate	10 mmol phosphate in 500 mL 0.9% w/v sodium chloride over 12 hours	Check salt used for other electrolyte content (see Appendix 2). May require special ordering if potassium content of salt used counts as high-strength. May be given peripherally depending on veins. More limited replacement would be 5 mmol in 250 ml 0.9% w/v sodium chloride over 6 hours. Higher concentrations should be administered centrally

* Any additions to fluid bags must be thoroughly mixed but preferably use commercial premixed bags or make in Technical Services (see Chapter 15).

† Caution is required in some patients, e.g. those with renal compromise.

Table 8.5 Typical oral or enteral electrolyte replacement to be modified according to local policy and patient's clinical condition*†

Electrolyte	Administration	Notes
Potassium	25–100 mmol/day, for example 2–8 Sando-K per day in divided doses (12 mmol potassium per tablet)	Use effervescent preparations rather than slow-release preparations
Magnesium	Up to 24 mmol/day in divided doses, for example magnesium glycerophosphate EP tablets (4 mmol or 97.2 mg magnesium per tablet) or magnesium oxide tablets 160–320 mg twice daily	Magnesium glycerophosphate tablets are unlicensed
Calcium	Up to 25 mmol/day	Not usually necessary or appropriate for nutritional patients unless already prescribed; consider intravenous supplementation instead
Phosphate	Up to 100 mmol in divided doses, for example Phosphate-Sandoz 3–6 tablets per day in divided doses (usually twice to four times a day)	Phosphate-Sandoz contains 16.1 mmol phosphate but also 20.4 mmol sodium and 3.1 mmol potassium per tablet

* Caution is required in some patients, e.g. those with renal compromise.
† Requires regular review.

Chapter 15). Furthermore, the bag may not even be administered (e.g. due to loss of appropriate intravenous access or suspected line sepsis). Notes on specific intravenous electrolyte replacement are shown in Table 8.4.

Any rapid electrolyte replacement may require electrocardiogram monitoring and repeated checks on blood levels, via either the biochemistry laboratory or a blood gas analyser. Repeat administration may be required before or after resampling for electrolyte levels.

Oral or enteral tube replacement of electrolytes is indicated when replacement is needed but when it is not necessary to use the intravenous route (i.e. when the gut is accessible and functioning). The quantity of an electrolyte administered via the oral or enteral tube route is almost always different to the intravenous route (Table 8.5), since administration into the gut requires absorption, which may be incomplete and takes time.

The use of enteral feeding tubes for electrolyte replacement can result in tube blockage from component interactions such as precipitation (see Chapter 5).

Although it is usually possible to add sodium or potassium to enteral feeds without adverse effects, never make additions of magnesium, calcium or phosphate which interact with enteral feeds as well as drugs. If you must prescribe magnesium, calcium or phosphate through an enteral feeding tube which is also used for enteral feeding, the feed must be discontinued approximately 2 hours before and not restarted until approximately 1 hour after the electrolyte administration and needs adequate flushing to limit local precipitation. Phosphate will precipitate with either calcium or magnesium and so concurrent administration of products containing these electrolytes is not possible. If absolutely necessary, leave a 1–2-hour gap with adequate tube flushing.

Specific electrolyte correction on high-care and intensive care units

High-care wards and intensive care units often have facilities that allow closer patient monitoring and nursing staff who are allowed to administer bolus doses of intravenous electrolytes in response to laboratory or blood gas results. It is therefore useful to consider the level of nursing input available to manage any serum electrolyte abnormalities since you may be able to be more cautious with electrolyte additions to the IVN if the ward can easily 'top up' low levels as required. However, even if the nursing staff can administer electrolytes in response to reported plasma levels, they will appreciate appropriate electrolyte additions to the IVN to avoid the need for repeated supplemental infusions.

Practical issues in electrolyte prescribing

Although ideally you will always have a complete set of electrolyte results (including recent trends) to support prescribing decisions, this is not always the case. You may therefore need to make judgements based on more limited information.

Unavailability of results

You must not assume that *all* electrolyte levels are normal when you have normal results for some, e.g. normal sodium, potassium and magnesium do not necessarily mean that there are no problems with phosphate levels. If a full set of electrolyte and renal function results are not available, some should be obtained as quickly as possible and IVN should not usually be prescribed until the results have been seen, since the risks of inappropriate electrolyte provision far outweigh the potential benefit from earlier IVN.

Nevertheless, it is sometimes possible to prescribe IVN safely in the absence of a complete set of electrolytes, providing those available are correctly interpreted in the context of the patient's clinical condition and the IVN energy and nitrogen are carefully prescribed as well as the electrolyte content. To do this you need to consider the patient's status and any available blood results to try to judge what the results might be had they been taken and whether they are likely to be rising or falling and how significant this change might be.

For example, the patient's renal function results are available and there is nothing to suggest renal compromise or worsening kidney function and the patient's available electrolytes are within normal trends and no other clinical factors indicate otherwise, standard quantities of magnesium and phosphate may be prescribed in the IVN. This would include making any allowances for likely deficiency or abnormal losses.

Chronic renal compromise without electrolyte retention will allow standard quantities of potassium, magnesium and phosphate to be included in your IVN prescription. If renal compromise is resulting in electrolyte retention and the serum potassium is towards (or above) the upper limit of the reference range, caution is indicated; a reduction in the potassium, magnesium and phosphate from standard in the IVN is likely to be appropriate. Additional supplemental electrolytes (beyond those in the IVN) can then be given if necessary once new plasma results are available, although this may result in unwanted fluid provision. In all cases where limited electrolytes are added to the IVN, remember that the refeeding syndrome remains a risk (see above and Chapter 9).

Timing results

Results from each day's blood samples usually take a few hours to become available and so you often need to base daily prescribing decisions on results from the previous day. Furthermore, patients can be clinically unstable and your regimen may run for up to 48 hours. It is therefore possible for clinical status to change and render the IVN electrolyte content of a regimen inappropriate for the patient (Figure 8.5). The problem can be even worse when prescribing in advance (e.g. at weekends).

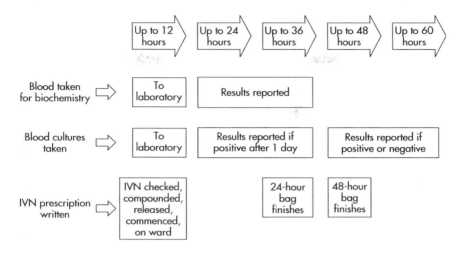

Figure 8.5 Typical timescales for laboratory reporting and administration of intravenous nutrition regimens.

Changing clinical circumstances

Although you should always try to avoid 'chasing your tail' with prescribing decisions, there are occasions when you will be faced with rapidly changing clinical circumstances that warrant a change in the IVN prescription when you only have a previously prescribed and compounded bag at your disposal. For example, the patient may require a reduction in the prescribed electrolytes in response to an unexpected upward trend in plasma levels (e.g. in acute prerenal failure). In this scenario, if another bag cannot be compounded, you need to consider modifying the rate of IVN infusion or changing any plans for additional infusions. Keeping your IVN prescribing as generally consistent as possible is helpful in all circumstances, so that whenever a previously compounded bag cannot be used in a patient, it can be utilised for another case. This limits financial waste and the unnecessary use of Technical Services' resources (see Chapter 15).

References

1. Wyeth Pharmaceuticals. Tazocin user leaflet section 4.4. Date of partial revision of the text 2 March 2005. Maidenhead: Wyeth Pharmaceuticals, 2005.
2. British Medical Association and the Royal Pharmaceutical Society of Great Britain. *British National Formulary* 36. London: British Medical Association and the Royal Pharmaceutical Society of Great Britain, 1998.

3. Association of the British Pharmaceutical Industry (2006). http://www.medicines.org.uk/ (accessed 11 June 2006).

4. Dukes M, Aronson J, eds. *Meyler's Side Effects of Drugs*, 14th edn. Amsterdam: Elsevier Science, 2000.

5. Davies D, Ferner R, de Glanville H, eds. *Davies's Textbook of Adverse Drug Reactions*, 5th edn. London: Chapman and Hall, 1998.

6. Evans D. *Special Tests: The Procedure and Meaning of the Commoner Tests in Hospital*. Bristol: J W Arrowsmith: 93.

7. Dukes M, Aronson J, eds. *Meyler's Side Effects of Drugs*. Oxford: Elsevier, 2000: 924–925.

8. Hayek M, Eisenberg P. Severe hypophosphataemia following the institution of enteral feedings. *Arch Surg* 1989; 124: 1325–1328.

9. Solomon S, Kirby D. The refeeding syndrome: a review. *J Parenteral Enteral Nutr* 1990; 14: 90–97.

10. Stryer L. *Biochemistry*, 4th edn. New York: W. H. Freeman, 1995: 310–311.

11. Lobo D, Bostock K, Neal K *et al*. Effect of salt and water balance on recovery of gastrointestinal function after elective colonic resection: a randomised controlled trial. *Lancet* 2002; 359: 1812–1818.

12. Brandstrup B, Tonnesen H, Beier-Holgersen R *et al*. Effects of intravenous fluid restriction on postoperative complications: comparison of two peri-operative fluid regimens: a randomized assessor-blinded multicenter trial. *Ann Surg* 2003; 238: 641–648.

13. Canary C, Guenter P, Love G *et al*. *Fluids and Electrolytes Made Incredibly Easy!* 2nd edn. Pennsylvania: Springhouse, 2002: 102.

14. Walker R, Edwards C, eds. *Clinical Pharmacy and Therapeutics*. London: Churchill Livingstone, 2003: 51–53.

15. Pennington C, ed. *Current Perspectives on Parenteral Nutrition in Adults: A Report by a Working Party of the British Association for Parenteral and Enteral Nutrition*. Maidenhead: British Association of Parenteral and Enteral Nutrition, 1996: 12–13.

16. Payne R, Little A, Williams R, Milner J. Interpretation of serum calcium in patients with abnormal serum proteins. *Br Med J* 1973; 4: 643–646.

17. Canary C, Guenter P, Love G *et al*. *Fluids and Electrolytes Made Incredibly Easy!* 2nd edn. Pennsylvania: Springhouse, 2002: 144–146.

18. Warrell D, Cox T, Firth J, Benz E, eds. *Oxford Textbook of Medicine*, 4th edn, vol. 3. Oxford: Oxford University Press, 2003: 160.

19. British Medical Association and the Royal Pharmaceutical Society of Great Britain. *British National Formulary* 49. London: British Medical Association and the Royal Pharmaceutical Society of Great Britain, 2005: 472.

20. NICE and the National Collaborating Centre For Acute Care. *Nutrition Support in Adults: Oral Nutrition Support, Enteral Tube Feeding and Parenteral Nutrition*. London: NICE and the National Collaborating Centre For Acute Care, 2006.

9

Micronutrients

Introduction

Micronutrients include vitamins, metals and trace elements. They have a wide variety of important roles, not least the facilitation of many processes that utilise or assimilate macronutrients from the diet or nutrition support. Although it is relatively unusual to see full-blown vitamin-deficiency states in the UK, iron deficiency is very common and it is not unusual to see the red, sore tongue of glossitis (suggestive of vitamin B-group deficiencies; Plate 3a) or the hypertrophied bleeding gums of scurvy (vitamin C depletion). Indeed, it is likely that most patients referred for intravenous nutrition (IVN) will be depleted in micronutrients to some extent and many will also have abnormally high demands or excessive losses. Since micronutrient depletion can result in clinical compromise, it is concerning that many IVN prescribers do not fully appreciate their importance and that Technical Services compounding units do not always ensure adequate provision in *all* IVN regimens. Indeed, a 2003 audit reported that one-third of patients did not receive correct levels of micronutrient additions despite nutritional assessment[1]. This is not only poor practice but is potentially dangerous and it goes against recommendations from the National Institute for Health and Clinical Excellence (NICE) (Box 9.1).

Since the mechanisms of micronutrient action and the consequences of their depletion are complex, this chapter does not attempt to cover them in detail. Instead it gives a broad outline of:

- The roles of micronutrients
- The causes of micronutrient depletion

Box 9.1 National Institute for Health and Clinical Excellence (NICE) recommendations on micronutrients and completeness of feeds[2]

'Always add micronutrients and trace elements to parenteral nutrition . . .'

- The consequences of micronutrient depletion
- The principles of micronutrient prescribing
- The likely levels of micronutrients needed in IVN regimens

The aim is for you to understand why all IVN regimens should be complete in micronutrients, who may need extra levels of supplementation and how you can best provide all requirements.

Causes and consequences of micronutrient depletion

Patients needing IVN are likely to be micronutrient-depleted due to:

- Poor long-term diets or insufficient recent intake
- Inadequate gastrointestinal absorption or excessive gastrointestinal losses
- Abnormalities in vitamin storage, processing or metabolic demands
- The effects of alcohol and other drugs

Furthermore, for those patients who have already started IVN or any other means of nutrition support, pre-existing depletion may be exacerbated by the arrival of macronutrients without an adequate micronutrient supply (refeeding effects). Similarly, the provision of some, but not all, micronutrients can lead to paradoxical depletion in other micronutrients.

Poor customary diet

Many individuals consume a diet with low micronutrient content. In some, it is simply a consequence of their eating 'junk food' with little fruit and vegetable intake. In others it is due to cultural dietary restriction such as those followed by vegans. There are also groups, particularly the elderly housebound, who simply eat very little food because their energy requirements are low and although this low intake may meet their energy and nitrogen demands, it may fall short in terms of adequate vitamins, minerals and trace element provision.

The most recent UK *National Diet and Nutrition Survey* confirmed that vitamin deficiencies are frequent, especially in the elderly. Low folate levels were found in 29% of those aged > 65 years living at home and low vitamin C in 14%. In nursing homes, the figures were even worse, rising to 40% and 35% respectively[3]. In addition, studies evaluating folate, vitamin B_{12} or vitamin B_6 deficiency on the basis of hyperhomocysteinaemia (a reversible marker of functional depletion: see below) demonstrated inadequate levels of one or more of these vitamins in 63% of apparently healthy older adults[4].

Insufficient recent intake due to illness or injury

As described in Chapter 4, the majority of patients referred for IVN have had little or no recent nutrient intake. As a consequence, they are at risk of multiple micronutrient deficiencies, particularly of the water-soluble group which have relatively limited body stores, e.g. some of the vitamin B group and vitamin C.

Poor absorption and excessive losses of micronutrients

In addition to poor nutrient intake, many IVN patients have limited absorptive capacity or abnormal losses. Patients with long-standing malabsorption due to conditions such as Crohn's disease (especially if they have had surgical resections) or coeliac disease are at clearest risk but most other IVN patients also have gastrointestinal function problems that have been developing for some time. Loss of jejunal function limits iron and water-soluble vitamin absorption whereas the more common loss of ileal function limits absorption of the fat-soluble vitamins A, D, E and K. The absorption of fat-soluble vitamins may also be compromised by jaundice or pancreatic disease and, although body stores are usually large, rapid depletion can occur if patients have significant bile salt losses (e.g. those with biliary drains or high-gut stomas). Limited absorption of fat-soluble vitamins has also been reported with low protein and zinc intakes[5].

Abnormal vitamin storage, processing, production and demands

Many IVN patients have problems that affect storage, processing, production and demands for micronutrients. Some of these are relatively specific, such as damage to either renal or liver function leading to decreased activation of vitamin D, with levels of vitamin D often low anyway in patients who are ill for long periods since the primary source is not intake but skin synthesis dependent on exposure to sunlight. Less specific micronutrient problems due to abnormal storage, metabolism or demands are probably even more widespread but less well characterised. For example, problems with liver function can compromise the status of numerous vitamins usually stored or processed there and systemic illness itself increases oxidative stresses and hence raises demands for antioxidant protection, including demands for vitamins A, C and E and trace elements such as zinc and selenium. Pregnant or breast-feeding women also have abnormally high micronutrient demands and turnover[6], although care must be taken, e.g. vitamin A is teratogenic in a high enough dose.

Alcohol and drug effects

Alcoholics are frequently micronutrient-depleted for several reasons. Almost all alcoholics eat poorly and many vomit or have poor small-bowel absorptive capacity (due to direct alcohol toxicity). If their liver is affected, they may also have vitamin-processing and storage problems and alcohol promotes increased renal micronutrient excretion in some cases, including thiamine. Although the most common deficiencies present in alcoholics are folate and vitamin C, the most clinically important is thiamine because of the dangers of Wernicke–Korsakoff syndrome triggered by refeeding (see below).

Some drugs can have direct effects on micronutrient levels, e.g. sodium valproate[7], whereas others can have indirect effects, e.g. antibiotics reducing the gut flora that produce vitamin K.

Refeeding effects

The need for micronutrient cofactors in the utilisation of protein, fat and carbohydrate means that their availability in adequate amounts is essential for the proper utilisation and assimilation of macronutrients in IVN. Of even more importance, however, is that provision of macronutrients without adequate micronutrients can precipitate a worsening of any pre-existing micronutrient deficiency since the delivery of the macronutrients will increase demands for the vitamins and trace elements involved in their metabolism. The most obvious example of this type of refeeding phenomenon is the Wernicke–Korsakoff syndrome in which neurological damage can occur from the acute worsening of thiamine depletion precipitated by nutrition support or even glucose administered without adequate thiamine cover to permit increased carbohydrate metabolism. However, it is very likely that other less clinically obvious refeeding phenomena of this type also occur. Indeed, these types of problem may contribute to the poor clinical outcomes seen when sick, depleted patients are given early, overenthusiastic nutrition support.

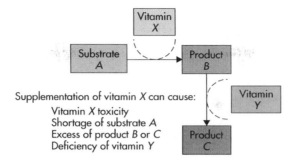

Figure 9.1 Consequences of unbalanced micronutrient provision.

Unbalanced micronutrient provision

Giving either a single micronutrient or a limited range of micronutrients, especially in large doses, can also cause problems. The reasons for this are varied but include direct toxicity from high dose, e.g. vitamin A is hepatotoxic in large amounts, and problems related to the functional effects of micronutrients when they 'overdrive' metabolic pathways. This can then deplete substrates for those pathways, generate excess products or precipitate secondary micronutrient deficiencies. This concept is shown in Figure 9.1.

A prime example of this type of problem is the interaction between vitamin B_{12} and folate in which administration of one can lead to profound depletion of the other.

Consequences of micronutrient depletion

The existence and importance of micronutrients were first appreciated through recognition of clinical deficiency states. For example, the existence of scurvy was initially linked to diets low in fresh fruit and vegetables aboard ships on long voyages. This then led to the later identification of vitamin C. However, although this type of thought process was crucial in developing concepts of vitamins and essential micronutrients, it has also led to widespread misunderstandings. Many health professionals still believe that the primary purpose of vitamins is to prevent the associated clinical deficiency state. Consequently, unless a patient has signs of scurvy, they believe that he or she is unlikely to be deficient in vitamin C. Similarly, patients with no retinal problems must have adequate vitamin A, and those without macrocytic anaemia cannot be short of vitamin B_{12} or folate. This is not necessarily the case. In reality, most vitamins have numerous different functions that are only just beginning to be understood. It therefore seems likely that many IVN patients may be suffering from some consequences of micronutrient shortages, even if they have no definite clinical symptoms or signs.

General consequences of depletion

Well before depletion of a micronutrient reaches levels at which clinical deficiency states are seen, some metabolic processes and physiological functions can be compromised. The concept is shown in Figure 9.2.

An example of vitamin depletion causing biochemical compromise before becoming clinically evident is found in studies of elevated homo-cysteine. The vitamins B_6, B_{12} and folate are all required by the liver to undertake transamination reactions. These move amine groups between different amino acid skeletons to synthesise amino acids that the body requires from those that are currently available. If one or more of these vitamins is not present in adequate amounts, the transamination reactions cannot be performed properly and instead some amino acid metabolism is diverted into the formation of homocysteine and other waste metabolites. High levels of homocysteine are generally considered to be toxic to the vasculature. In a study conducted by Joosten *et al.*, high levels were seen in 63% of healthy over-65-year-olds and 83% of the elderly in hospital[4]. Furthermore, the study showed that the raised

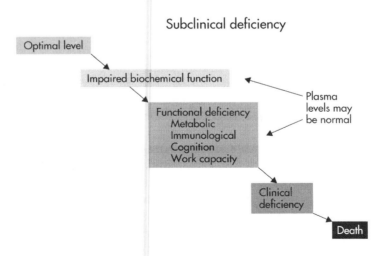

Figure 9.2 The severity of micronutrient depletion determines the resulting effects.

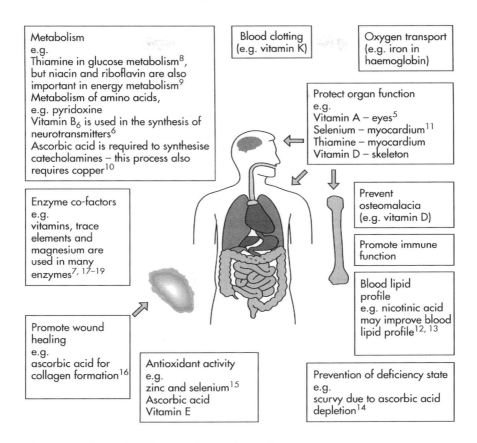

Metabolism
e.g.
Thiamine in glucose metabolism[8],
but niacin and riboflavin are also
important in energy metabolism[9]
Metabolism of amino acids,
e.g. pyridoxine
Vitamin B_6 is used in the synthesis of
neurotransmitters[6]
Ascorbic acid is required to synthesise
catecholamines – this process also
requires copper[10]

Blood clotting
(e.g. vitamin K)

Oxygen transport
(e.g. iron in
haemoglobin)

Protect organ function
e.g.
Vitamin A – eyes[5]
Selenium – myocardium[11]
Thiamine – myocardium
Vitamin D – skeleton

Enzyme co-factors
e.g.
vitamins, trace
elements and
magnesium are
used in many
enzymes[7, 17–19]

Prevent
osteomalacia
(e.g. vitamin D)

Promote immune
function

Blood lipid
profile
e.g. nicotinic acid
may improve blood
lipid profile[12, 13]

Promote wound
healing
e.g.
ascorbic acid for
collagen formation[16]

Antioxidant activity
e.g.
zinc and selenium[15]
Ascorbic acid
Vitamin E

Prevention of deficiency state
e.g.
scurvy due to ascorbic acid
depletion[14]

Figure 9.3 Examples of some micronutrient roles.

levels were reduced by vitamin supplementation to levels seen in healthy young adults. These results suggests that functional vitamin B_6, vitamin B_{12} or folate deficiency is very common and may be present in subjects with normal plasma vitamin levels and bone marrow function.

Discussions of this type make definition of all the different vitamins' roles very difficult since every one has multiple functions. Figure 9.3 should therefore be viewed as an illustration of just some of the micronutrient actions although, in reality, many more processes will not work at full capacity if deficiencies are present. It also seems likely that micronutrient deficiency effects will limit clinical progress in the multiply-depleted IVN patient. It is for this reason, along with the refeeding dangers noted above, that we advocate addition of micro-nutrients to *all* IVN regimens.

Specific micronutrient deficiency states and dangers of micronutrient toxicity

Although micronutrients should not be thought of as solely acting to prevent the described deficiency states, all IVN prescribers should still be able to recognise those states and should be aware of patients who are at specific risk of depletion. Furthermore, they should know of the potential adverse effects of excessive specific supplementation.

Vitamin A

Most people know of the link between vitamin A deficiency and visual problems, especially night blindness. This is rarely seen in the UK, except in patients with very severe fat malabsorption, such as those with extensive ileal resection or chronic pancreatic insufficiency (including patients with cystic fibrosis). Worldwide, however, dietary vitamin A deficiency is common and depletion at levels that do not cause retinal problems still leads to vulnerability to measles and gastrointestinal or respiratory infections. Furthermore, vitamin A supplementation reduces mortality from these conditions by more than 50%[20]. It therefore seems likely that adequate provision of vitamin A in IVN is helpful to some IVN patients, especially those who have had prolonged periods of inadequate intake or those who may have become rapidly depleted in vitamin A through excess bile salt loss.

Vitamin A in excess is a potent cause of liver damage and patients with liver disease may be particularly vulnerable. It is therefore essential that any provision at levels above those recommended for maintenance are only used for limited periods, especially as measured levels are difficult to interpret without accounting for changes in retinol-binding protein, to which the vitamin is bound (see below).

Vitamin C

Overt vitamin C depletion (scurvy) is seen in UK clinical practice, especially in alcoholics, patients with severe anorexia nervosa and those with long-term gastrointestinal disease with malabsorption. It typically causes gum hypertrophy and inflammation, loss of teeth and skin rashes, including a haemorrhagic rash around hair follicles on the legs. Once again, you need to be aware that even without overt scurvy, depletion of vitamin C can probably compromise wound healing and may limit antioxidant defences. It is therefore an essential component in all IVN regimens. Vitamin C toxicity does not seem to be a problem.

Vitamin D

Significant vitamin D deficiency is also seen in the UK although its manifestations are harder to identify. Rickets with skeletal deformity and abnormal gait does occur but is unusual since deficiency has to be profound and rickets only occurs in children. Adults get osteomalacia, which may present with fracture but more frequently causes pelvic bone pain, coupled with aching muscles and general weakness (particularly in the legs). More commonly still, osteomalacia is a biochemical diagnosis, suspected from low plasma calcium and alkaline phosphatase measurements found by chance. These are then confirmed by low measures of vitamin D. Osteomalacia usually occurs in patients who have either overt malnutrition or fat absorption problems, or those who have very little skin exposure to sunlight. Patients with chronic renal or liver disease are also at risk of vitamin D deficiency since activation depends on two hydroxylation steps that occur sequentially in those organs.

Vitamin D in excess can cause hypercalcaemia and risks metastatic calcification or pseudogout. Monitoring plasma calcium levels is mandatory if giving high-dose, specific replacement of vitamin D rather than maintenance-level supplementation.

Vitamin E

The lipid-soluble vitamin E plays a role in antioxidant and immune system defences. Deficiency, for example in malabsorption due to Crohn's[21], can cause neuropathy and myopathy, although even without overt deficiency, depletion may impair immunity and potentially compromise the patient. Status needs to be interpreted in the context of a lipid profile because vitamin E is carried on lipoproteins in the plasma and hence apparently low levels may be due to abnormal lipid profiles rather than genuine deficiency.

Vitamin B$_1$ (thiamine)

Severe thiamine deficiency is perhaps the most common real micronutrient threat to IVN patients[8,22]. As mentioned above, the arrival of macronutrients in individuals with micronutrient depletion can worsen the situation by increasing demands for them. In the case of thiamine it is the needs of carbohydrate metabolism that precipitate acute further deficiency problems that can be manifest as the Wernicke–Korsakoff syndrome (Wernicke's encephalopathy). Features are shown in Box 9.2.

Box 9.2 Features of Wernicke–Korsakoff syndrome

Memory loss
Loss of muscle co-ordination
Double vision
Disorders of eye movement
Confabulation
Hallucinations
Amnesia
Psychosis

Beriberi with cardiac failure and peripheral neuropathy is also a conequence of thiamine depletion. It probably occurs less commonly than the Wernicke–Korsakoff syndrome but can go unrecognised since poor cardiac function is easily ascribed to other problems such as sepsis and multiorgan failure. The possibility that cardiac failure in a malnourished IVN patient might be due to thiamine depletion is therefore rarely considered.

Almost any patient referred for IVN is at some risk of thiamine deficiency since body stores are low and are quickly depleted. As discussed above, those with high alcohol intakes are at particular risk but it is essential that *all* patients needing IVN are never prescribed it without thiamine. Thiamine toxicity with headaches, irritability, insomnia and weakness can occur but doses of more than 3 g/day are probably needed to induce such effects.

Vitamin B$_2$ (riboflavin)

Riboflavin is needed for the metabolism of carbohydrate, fat and amino acids and so, once again, should be an integral part of IVN provision. Deficiency usually manifests as a sore mouth, tongue and lips and is particularly seen in vegans. Toxicity does not seem to be a problem.

Vitamin B$_3$ (nicotinic acid or niacin)

Nicotinic acid deficiency causes pellagra – a condition comprising dermatitis, diarrhoea, fatigue, insomnia and dementia. It can be fatal. It is most commonly seen in alcoholics or those with long-term malabsorption problems. High doses of nicotinic acid can cause skin irritation and rashes, and very high doses are toxic to the liver and kidney.

Vitamin B$_6$ (pyridoxine)

As described above, vitamin B$_6$ is needed for amino acid metabolism and IVN delivery of amino acids will increase demands. Deficiency causes stomatitis, glossitis, hypochromic anaemia and convulsions. Levels are also lowered by some drugs (e.g. penicillamine[23,24], oestrogen contraceptive pills[24] and long-term theophylline[24]). Toxicity is rare but can cause nerve damage.

Vitamin B$_{12}$ and folate

Deficiency of vitamin B$_{12}$ and/or folate is common. Low levels of either cause macrocytic anaemia, peripheral neuropathy and central nervous system damage. However, as noted above, lesser deficiency also compromises amino acid metabolism and probably has numerous other ill effects. Vitamin B$_{12}$ deficiency can occur in strict vegetarians and specific absorption problems are seen in Crohn's patients with terminal ileal disease, patients with pernicious anaemia and those postgastrectomy. Bacterial overgrowth can also utilise B$_{12}$ in the small bowel. Marginal folate deficiency from a poor diet is very common. No direct toxic effects from excessive B$_{12}$ or folate are likely.

Vitamin K

Vitamin K is mainly produced by gut bacteria and deficiency in the absence of gastrointestinal disease or related complications (e.g. obstruction of the bile duct) is unusual.

Vitamin K has an important role in blood clotting but is also involved in the metabolism of bone. Deficiency or antagonism of vitamin K leads to effects such as ready bleeding, skeletal deformities and deposition of calcium in the vasculature. Overzealous provision of vitamin K can lead to effects including difficulty achieving therapeutic effectiveness with oral anticoagulants (e.g. warfarin).

Vitamin K status can be assessed by the reported international normalised ratio (INR) unless liver disease compromises INR directly.

Biotin

Biotin deficiency, causing dermatitis, hair loss, glossitis, anorexia and depression, is very unusual but has been reported in patients on long-term IVN. Toxicity has not been reported.

Iron

Iron deficiency, usually due to gastrointestinal or perioperative blood loss, is seen extremely frequently in the IVN patient population. It causes anaemia, smooth glossitis (Plate 3b), angular cheilitis and nail damage. Iron is therefore an essential component in longer-term IVN provision. In the shorter term, however, the provision of intravenous iron to sick patients does raise concerns. Studies in famine situations show that iron supplementation, even orally, increases mortality. It is postulated that this is due to iron's stimulating effect on the growth of micro-organisms or an effect of promoting pro-oxidant, free-radical damage[25]. If either is the case, iron provision to the acutely unwell or septic patient may also have adverse effects, especially in surgical patients in whom tissue damage releases significant quantities of iron. We therefore recommend that specific iron supplementation is avoided in most acute IVN patients and that if patients are significantly iron-depleted, blood transfusion is used instead despite the inherent risks of that process.

Zinc

The perioral and perineal rash of zinc deficiency is not uncommon on intensive care units. Alcoholics or anorexia nervosa patients with super-imposed critical illness are particularly vulnerable but it is also seen in patients with long-standing severe gastrointestinal disease such as Crohn's. Zinc is required for innumerable enzymatic processes and is also required for gene transcription and cell replication. Adequate availability is therefore essential for the metabolism of protein, fat and carbohydrate and low levels will also impair wound healing and cause diarrhoea. Interestingly, zinc deficiency tends to cause marked anorexia and a striking change or loss in taste sensation[26]. This leads patients with marginal zinc status to describe food as tasting of metal or cardboard. Deficiency can also lead to crinkly hair growth and so it is sometimes possible to make a fairly confident diagnosis of zinc deficiency on clinical grounds.

In view of the above, it is clear that IVN should not be administered without adequate zinc being present. Toxicity only occurs with high doses for prolonged periods but must be borne in mind if using specific zinc supplements to promote wound healing (see below). Acute toxicity causes nausea and vomiting whereas chronic overadministration causes secondary copper deficiency with microcytic anaemia and neutropenia.

Copper

Like zinc, copper is an essential component of many metalloenzymes but deficiency is probably rare. Nevertheless, it should be suspected in cases of microcytic anaemia that fail to respond to iron supplementation, particularly if there is also neutropenia and the patient is very malnourished. Toxicity is very unlikely but causes widespread tissue damage (as seen in Wilson's disease, when an abnormality of metabolism leads to copper excess). Copper is primarily excreted via the bile and so particular care must be taken in patients with disturbance of normal bile metabolism. Patients who have biliary obstruction are prone to developing high levels of copper when it is provided for long periods within IVN, whereas those who have excessive bile losses through biliary drains or high-gut stomas may develop copper-deficiency states surprisingly quickly.

Selenium

Selenium is an important component of enzymes involved in antioxidant protection. It is therefore likely that IVN patients have relatively high demands and so it is logical to provide generous quantities to potentially depleted IVN patients. This applies especially early in their clinical course. Excessive selenium administration can result in adverse effects, including hair loss, 'garlic breath', nail changes and peripheral neuropathy[27].

Manganese

Manganese is required for many enzymes and deficiency can cause problems such as anaemia and lipid abnormalities. However, it is more frequent to encounter problems of excess manganese provision in patients on long-term IVN support which can result in neurological damage. Like copper, manganese is excreted via bile and so particular care is needed to avoid overprovision in patients with compromised biliary drainage.

Measuring micronutrient status

All hospitals can provide measurements of iron status, vitamin B_{12}, folate and vitamin D. Many can also measure vitamin A and E and some will assay trace elements, usually providing levels for zinc, selenium, copper and manganese. Results, however, are usually slow to come back and their interpretation is difficult due to:

- Relevance of plasma levels to intracellular tissue levels
- Acute-phase effects on binding proteins, e.g. iron and transferrin, vitamin A and retinol-binding protein, zinc and albumin, copper and caeruloplasmin
- Leakage from the liver, e.g. vitamin B_{12}
- Effects of other plasma components, e.g. vitamin E levels with lipid levels (see above)
- Interactions of micronutrient deficiencies

In view of these difficulties, your practice will often need to be pragmatic – provide all micronutrients generously anyway and only make adjustments if measurements reveal very high or very low specific levels. Baseline measurements should probably be made in patients who are likely to require longer-term IVN with follow-up monitoring if this proves to be the case. Whenever taking blood for trace element analysis, special trace-element-free tubes are required to prevent sample contamination.

Principles and practice of micronutrient prescribing

The aim of IVN prescribing is to ensure that your regimen meets all of your patient's needs. From the information given above, it is possible to draw up some principles governing your prescription so that:

- You do not give IVN without full micronutrient provision.
- You provide generous micronutrient supplementation during the early phase of IVN while avoiding excess provision of micronutrients that might encourage microbial growth or increase free-radical damage.
- You give additional, specific vitamin supplementation to patients with overt deficiency states or at high risk of specific deficiencies.

However, before deciding on appropriate levels of micronutrient provision, you must assess inputs from other sources by checking oral intake, drug charts and other intravenous prescriptions.

Non-intravenous nutrition sources of micronutrients

Patients who can swallow and absorb nutrients may be on oral micronutrient preparations whereas others may be meeting some of their needs from diet, sip-feeds or enteral tube feeding. Nevertheless, since IVN is used in patients with intestinal failure or inaccessible gastrointestinal tracts, it is not usual for IVN patients to come even close to meeting their micronutrient needs from oral or enteral routes. Furthermore, many oral multivitamin preparations lack some vitamins or trace elements and, although sip-feeds and enteral feeds usually contain all necessary micronutrients, they only deliver the daily recommended nutrient intake (RNI) of every micronutrient when patients are meeting their full energy needs from that product. Sometimes specific individual vitamins are given by mouth, e.g. oral thiamine in known alcoholics.

Some patients are receiving or have received micronutrients by the intramuscular or intravenous routes. For example, Pabrinex may have been given to alcoholics and many patients with terminal ileal dysfunction are on intramuscular vitamin B_{12} supplements.

Principle 1: Do not give intravenous nutrition without full micronutrient provision

Providing IVN without the addition of micronutrients can precipitate dangerous refeeding problems and may limit full utilisation and metabolism of the macronutrients. Since you have no way of knowing which micronutrient levels are compromised, a balance of all micronutrients should be given. In our opinion, and that of NICE (Box 9.1), measures to ensure that IVN is not started 'out of hours' without appropriate micronutrient additions are essential (see Chapter 16).

Principle 2: Provide generous micronutrient supplementation during the early phase of intravenous nutrition while avoiding excess provision of micronutrients that may encourage microbial growth or increase free-radical damage

During the initial provision of IVN, levels of vitamins and trace elements provided to most patients should probably be greater than those needed to maintain health since you may need to replenish existing deficiency as well as meet exceptional demands and maximise antioxidant capabilities. This concept is shown in Figure 9.4.

The standard recommendations for micronutrient provision in IVN, and hence most dose units, are set to meet normal demands and daily requirements. However, we recommend that higher levels of vitamins, aiming to give about twice the 'normal' daily requirements, should be used during the first 10–14 days of IVN, with the aim of replenishing depleted stores while meeting excessive demands. This level should pose no significant risk of toxicity.

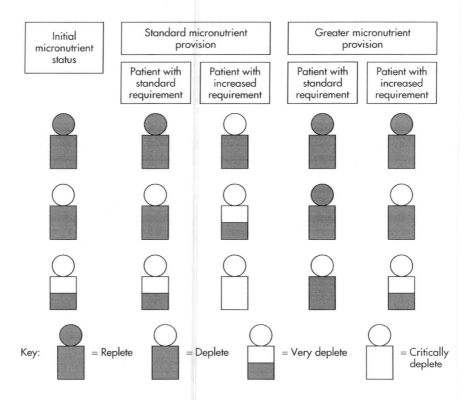

Figure 9.4 Consider increased provision of micronutrients in patients likely to be deplete.

Prescribing double the standard trace element additives should also be useful but may, depending on the product used, increase the provision of iron and copper, which could have adverse effects on microbial growth and free-radical damage. We therefore recommend that, during early IVN, especially in acutely injured or septic patients, double daily quantities of zinc and selenium are provided and no extra iron or copper is given. Following this repletion period, prescribing should be amended to provide normal maintenance levels.

Principle 3: Give additional, specific vitamin supplementation to patients with overt deficiency states or those at very high risk of specific deficiencies

Patients with overt signs of vitamin deficiency or those with measurably low levels of individual micronutrients (accounting for the likely effects of any acute-phase response on reported levels) will need either specific additions to their IVN or additional supplementation. Higher levels of thiamine should be given to all those at high risk of refeeding syndrome and specific additions of other vitamins are also appropriate for heavy drinkers, especially those with alcoholic liver disease, the elderly and those with non-healing wounds. If giving extra micronutrients, you must be aware, as with all other IVN additions, of any stability issues before prescribing (see Appendix 1). Generally, the addition of water-soluble vitamins is not likely to cause problems although the addition of lipid-soluble vitamins may well cause solubility concerns.

Risks of refeeding syndrome

Patients at very high risk of the electrolyte and fluid disturbances of refeeding syndrome (see Chapter 8) are also likely to have significant thiamine depletion. Intravenous Pabrinex, 1 pair of ampoules once a day for 3 days, in addition to your standard micronutrient additives, should provide enough thiamine to avoid problems. Before prescribing check for any previous allergic reaction to Pabrinex or any other micronutrient supplementation. Pabrinex can be added to the IVN following confirmation of adequate stability or run separately over the recommended duration.

Elderly patients

The Joosten study described above[4] showed that hospitalised patients over 65 years of age are very likely to be deficient in vitamin B_{12} or folate. We therefore suggest that additional specific replacement should be given. Do not prescribe either vitamin B_{12} or folic acid alone, since a deficiency of one can be masked or uncovered by provision of the other. Suitable replacement of vitamin B_{12} and folic acid for patients over 65 years of age comprises:

- 1 mg vitamin B_{12} once a day for three doses, on either consecutive or alternative days. This can either be added to the IVN regimen or administered intramuscularly.
- Folic acid 5 mg daily – usually added to the IVN, although it can also be administered enterally or by separate intravenous infusion.

If a patient is to receive vitamin B_{12} in the IVN bags and is commencing at quarter-rate (see Chapter 7), give a total of four doses rather than the standard three to ensure adequate provision. Folic acid administration

---

Box 9.3 Micronutrients for non-healing wounds

Specific provision of:
Zinc
Vitamin B$_{12}$
Folic acid
Ascorbic acid

in addition to routine multivitamin and trace element provision – review every 7 days

Also consider twice-daily topical sunflower-seed oil if dry, fragile, flaking skin suggests essential fatty acid deficiency[28]

---

should be continued for 2–3 weeks, switching to oral or enteral administration if the patient has discontinued IVN after the vitamin B$_{12}$ doses.

Non-healing wounds

Micronutrients are important in the repair of wounds and a deficiency of some micronutrients results in poor wound healing. A patient with non-healing wounds, including chronic ulcers, may therefore benefit from specific micronutrient replacement, as shown in Box 9.3.

Prescribing micronutrients with abnormal reported levels

If the result of a micronutrient assay shows probable depletion (taking into account the difficulties in interpretation discussed above), it is usually appropriate to provide additional specific supplementation of that micronutrient for about 10–14 days before rechecking the level. High doses are not always necessary and daily maintenance quantities may correct deficits, particularly if there is some concurrent intake from oral or enteral routes. If the level remains low on rechecking, increased specific supplementation may be indicated, usually comprising two or three times 'normal' maintenance quantities.

If a level is raised but within two multiples of the upper limit of the reference range, simply recheck after 7–10 days. If the level remains high and especially if it is rising or the patient is pregnant or breast-feeding, caution is necessary and provision should be cut, followed by rechecking after 10–14 days.

Reducing provision of a specific micronutrient where you are using a preparation with a range of micronutrients usually requires the use of an alternative product unless you are also happy to reduce provision of the other micronutrients (possibly starting supplementation of specific other micronutrients). As a guide, reducing provision by a quarter to three-quarters, depending on how high the result is, is likely to be reasonable.

Practical aspects of micronutrient prescribing

There are many micronutrient products available for prescribing containing either one or more micronutrients. Examples of products suitable for IVN use are compared to the recommendations for provision from the British Association for Parenteral and Enteral Nutrition (BAPEN)[29] in Appendix 3.

Normal prescribing

Maintenance daily amounts of vitamins in IVN are usually achieved by prescribing 1 vial of Cernevit or 10 ml of Vitlipid Adult plus one vial of Solivito N daily. However, since we advocate a normal practice of giving twice the maintenance of vitamins during early feeding, twice these daily amounts need to be given for the first 10–14 days. Furthermore, since we also advocate that for most patients IVN should be started at a maximum of 50% of macronutrient requirements (see Chapter 7) and that this might best be achieved by running the first IVN regimen bag at half-rate, putting four times the standard daily recommendations into the first regimen would be ideal, followed by cutting to double standard quantities once the regimen is being given at full-rate. However, stability considerations usually limit additions to any bag to double daily maintenance requirements and, in all cases, we would recommend a reduction to the normal maintenance provision of intravenous micronutrients and trace elements after 10–14 days.

In very exceptional circumstances, IVN without additions but with concurrent Pabrinex and careful monitoring has been advocated but we would not recommend this practice (see Chapter 16).

Maintenance levels of trace elements usually come from 40 ml of Decan or 10 ml/day of Additrace. However, as noted above, doubling of these maintenance quantities would potentially be hazardous and so we prefer to give double maintenance quantities of zinc and selenium during the early part of IVN prescribing in sick patients, avoiding giving iron and copper. We therefore recommend 5 ml Multitrace 2 Plus or appropriate individual zinc and selenium additions. Double these quantities are needed in the first bag if run at quarter- or half-rate.

Guide to specific micronutrient supplementation

Appropriate doses for specific micronutrient supplementation always depend on the patient, but a guide to reasonable 'typical' doses is given in Appendix 3. Products for supplementation may be available in licensed form but, if not, consider unlicensed provision, taking into account product quality and reliability of the supplier. If specific micronutrient provision is indicated in a patient, it is likely that the patient will also be deficient in some other micronutrients. Such a patient should usually therefore also receive a complete micronutrient prescription providing a full range of vitamins and trace elements.

Duplication of micronutrient prescribing

Micronutrient supplementation via the oral or enteral tube route can usually be temporarily discontinued if the patient is receiving adequate quantities in the IVN and not doing so poses a risk of overdose. The exception is when patients need specific high-dose supplementation, for example pyridoxine-dependent epileptic seizures[30].

References

1. Newton R, Hardy G. British Pharmaceutical Nutrition Group/Hospital Pharmacists' Group (meeting report). *Hosp Pharm* 2004; 11: 346.
2. NICE and the National Collaborating Centre For Acute Care. *Nutrition Support in Adults: Oral Nutrition Support, Enteral Tube Feeding and Parenteral Nutrition*. London: NICE and the National Collaborating Centre For Acute Care, 2006.
3. Department of Health. *National Diet and Nutrition Survey: People Aged 65 Years and Over*. London: The Stationery Office, 1998.
4. Joosten E, van den Berg A, Riezler R *et al*. Metabolic evidence that deficiencies of vitamin B-12 (cobalamin), folate, and vitamin B-6 occur commonly in elderly people. *Am J Clin Nutr* 1993; 58: 468–476.
5. Spits Y, De Laey J, Leroy B. Rapid recovery of night blindness due to obesity surgery after vitamin A repletion therapy. *Br J Ophthalmol* 2004; 88: 583–585.
6. Schulze-Bonhage A, Kurthen M, Walger P, Elger C. Pharmacorefractory status epilepticus due to low vitamin B_6 levels during pregnancy. *Epilepsia* 2004; 45: 81–84.
7. Baggot P, Kalamarides J, Shoemaker J. Valproate-induced biochemical abnormalities in pregnancy corrected by vitamins: a case report. *Epilepsia* 1999; 40: 512–515.
8. Solomon S, Kirby D. The refeeding syndrome: a review. *J Parenteral Enteral Nutr* 1990; 14: 90–97.
9. Brody T. *Nutritional Biochemistry*, London: Academic Press, 1994: 355–357.

10. Brody T. *Nutritional Biochemistry*, 2nd edn. London: Academic Press, 1999: 623–624.
11. Payne-James, Grimble G, Silk D, eds. *Artificial Nutrition Support in Clinical Practice*, 2nd edn. London: Greenwich Medical Media, 2001: 195–196.
12. Brody T. *Nutritional Biochemistry*. London: Academic Press, 1994: 368–370.
13. British Medical Association and the Royal Pharmaceutical Society of Great Britain. *British National Formulary 36*. London: British Medical Association and the Royal Pharmaceutical Society of Great Britain, 1998: 120.
14. Kumar P, Clark M, eds. *Cinical Medicine*, 3rd edn. London: Bailliere Tindall, 1994: 164–165.
15. Sappey C, Leclercq P, Coudray C *et al*. Vitamin, trace element and peroxide status in HIV seropositive patients: asymptomatic patients present a severe, carotene deficiency. *Clin Chim Acta* 1994; 35–42.
16. Brody T. *Nutritional Biochemistry*. London: Academic Press, 1994: 621–623.
17. Brody T. *Nutritional Biochemistry*. London: Academic Press, 1994: 491.
18. Brody T. *Nutritional Biochemistry*. London: Academic Press, 1994: 795–796.
19. Payne-James J, Grimble G, Silk D, eds. *Artificial Nutrition Support in Clinical Practice*, 2nd edn. London: Greenwich Medical Media, 2001; 197–198.
20. Rahmathullah L, Underwood B, Thulasiraj R *et al*. Reduced mortality among children in southern India receiving a small weekly dose of vitamin A. *N Engl J Med* 1990; 323: 929–935.
21. Payne-James, Grimble G, Silk D, eds. *Artificial Nutrition Support in Clinical Practice*, 2nd edn. London: Greenwich Medical Media, 2001: 558–559.
22. Chadda K, Raynard B, Antoun S *et al*. Acute lactic acidosis with Wernicke's encephalopathy due to acute thiamine deficiency. *Intens Care Med* 2002; 28: 1499.
23. Dukes M, Aronson J, eds. *Meyler's Side Effects of Drugs*, 14th edn. Amsterdam: Elsevier Science, 2000: 723–727.
24. Davies D, Ferner R, de Glanville H, eds. *Davies's Textbook of Adverse Drug Reactions*, 5th edn. London: Chapman and Hall, 1998: 495–496.
25. Prescott L, Harley J, Klein D. *Microbiology*, 2nd edn. Oxford: Wm. C. Brown, 1993: 97–104.
26. Rang H, Dale M, Ritter J. *Pharmacology*, 3rd edn. London: Churchill Livingstone, 1995: 256–257.
27. Sweetman S, ed. *Martindale: The Complete Drug Reference*, 33rd edn. London: Pharmaceutical Press, 2002: 1375.
28. Sweetman S, ed. *Martindale: The Complete Drug Reference*, 33rd edn. London: Pharmaceutical Press, 2002: 1381.
29. Pennington C, ed. *Current Perspectives on Parenteral Nutrition in Adults: A Report by a Working Party of the British Association for Parenteral and Enteral Nutrition*. Maidenhead: British Association for Parenteral and Enteral Nutrition, 1996: 40–41.
30. Schulze-Bonhage A, Kurthen M, Walger P, Elger C. Pharmacorefractory status epilepticus due to low vitamin B_6 levels during pregnancy. *Epilepsia* 2004; 45: 81–84.

10

Prescribing for patients with specific problems

Introduction

Many intravenous nutrition (IVN) patients need special regimens because of problems with renal, liver, pancreatic, cardiac or respiratory function and some also have special needs related to specific types of gastrointestinal failure such as short-bowel syndrome (SBS) or high-output fistulae. Prescribing for these patients can be very specialised but the factors that need to be taken into consideration should be understood by all IVN prescribers.

Renal compromise

Many IVN patients have some degree of renal failure due to recent acute illness or injury, with consequent acute renal damage, or more specific acute or chronic renal disease. The medical notes should provide information on any known renal diagnosis and up-to-date biochemical results, especially recent changes, will indicate the level of current impairment.

Serum creatinine is used to measure kidney function because renal compromise limits the ability to excrete it, yet production from muscle is relatively constant. Causes of renal impairment are classified as:

- *Prerenal*: poor perfusion from causes such as dehydration, low blood pressure or renovascular disease
- *Renal*: intrinsic kidney disease such as diabetic nephropathy and glomerulonephritis
- *Postrenal*: obstruction of urine flow due to ureteric, bladder or postbladder problems

All three types of damage lead to raised creatinine, although levels must be interpreted accounting for a patient's muscle mass. In particular, malnourished patients with a low muscle mass produce relatively less creatinine than expected and hence significant renal impairment may not be associated with creatinine levels as high as those seen in normally nourished patients.

Plasma urea levels also rise with any form of renal impairment but are more sensitive to dehydration. A relatively greater rise in urea than creatinine therefore suggests that the patient is dry unless there is another reason for urea production levels to be raised. The latter is an issue in patients who have had a significant upper gastrointestinal bleed when high levels of digested protein (from blood in the upper gut) are delivered to the liver. As with creatinine, starving individuals with low muscle mass and low levels of protein intake and turnover may have lower urea levels than would be expected for any degree of renal function. Urea levels may also be low in patients with severe liver disease who are unable to synthesise urea even if faced with excessive protein delivery from an upper gastrointestinal bleed.

Prescribing IVN for patients with poor renal function often needs reduced levels of electrolytes and extreme care with fluid provision. The following considerations are therefore important:

- *Sodium in renal disease*: patients with renal damage can have problems with either sodium retention or excessive sodium loss. Any tendency to retain sodium often accompanies a tendency to retain fluid and similarly excessive sodium losses often accompany polyuria. However, these relationships are not universal and measuring urinary sodium levels in addition to blood levels is often very valuable (see Chapter 8). Clinical assessment of hydration status is also important.
- *Potassium*: renal impairment often leads to retention of potassium and the consequent need to reduce provision in IVN regimens. Review of previously prescribed potassium from all routes and any trends in plasma potassium levels helps to determine the severity of potassium retention and hence likely requirements. It is often easier and safer to prescribe regimens with no potassium and then provide any that is needed separately in order to gain flexibility and close control.
- *Fluid*: renal impairment often results in fluid retention and oliguria and you will need to liaise with ward clinicians to ensure that patients meet the necessary volume restriction. All fluid provision must be accounted for including that from the IVN, other intravenous fluids and intravenous drugs, and any oral or enteral intake. You may need to restrict IVN volume, although sometimes this can remain normal if other intravenous infusions and drug dilution

volumes can be reduced. During resolution of acute renal impairment and in some forms of chronic renal disease, polyuria is seen with losses of very large quantities of fluid and electrolytes. These must be tracked and met carefully in order to avoid a further dehydration insult or significant electrolyte loss, e.g. development of hypokalaemia. However, they should not be tracked so closely that any oedema resulting from previous oliguria is not permitted to resolve. It is not unusual to find oedematous patients with improving renal function receiving huge amounts of fluid because of prescribing to provide *'measured losses + 500 mL insensible'* which commenced when renal function was very poor.

- *Magnesium*: as with potassium, renal impairment often means that IVN provision of magnesium needs to be reduced or removed completely with separate, more flexible intravenous administration as necessary.
- *Calcium*: plasma calcium levels can be low in renal disease because of potential influences of hyperphosphataemia and decreased renal production of 1,25-hydroxycholecalciferol (activated vitamin D) which can limit calcium absorption and retention. However, they can also be high if too much is given (since renal clearance is poor) and in chronic renal impairment, initial compensatory changes causing low levels can then lead to high parathormone levels (secondary hyperparathyroidism) which can go on to become excessive with consequent hypercalcaemic problems (tertiary hyperparathyroidism). In view of the above processes, chronic renal failure can result in a number of bone mineralisation and density problems and excessive calcium replacement with hyperphosphataemia can result in metastatic calcification. Overall, patients with renal disease may therefore need anything from low to high calcium in their IVN regimen, and you will need to take into account current plasma calcium and phosphate levels and, in longer-term patients, measures of vitamin D, active vitamin D, parathormone and what is known about bone density (from dual-spectrum X-ray densitometry (DEXA) scanning; see Chapter 13).
- *Phosphate*: retention as a result of renal impairment usually requires a reduction in provision of phosphate in IVN regimens. Phosphate retention leading to hyperphosphataemia can lower the plasma ionised calcium.
- *Protein and energy in renal disease*: although traditionally patients with renal impairment were given reduced levels of protein in order to limit the production of urea and other nitrogenous metabolic

end-products, it has now been recognised that subnormal nitrogen provision will lead, in most patients, to greater breakdown of their own nitrogen stores with similar net production of urea and other metabolites. Current thinking therefore recommends 'standard' levels of protein provision and we too recommend this, taking into account the suggested restrictions on higher protein feeding which we believe may be harmful in very sick individuals (see Chapter 7). Energy provision should be generous (within the limits imposed by refeeding risks; see Chapter 7) to try to minimise endogenous protein breakdown and net lean tissue loss. However, in cases when renal failure is severe (e.g. a creatinine clearance of less than 30 mL/min) and the patient has symptomatic uraemia, restriction of protein provision may be helpful, although it may be more reasonable to maintain proper levels of feeding and to use dialysis or haemofiltration to reduce uraemia. If you are restricting protein content of IVN regimens, remember to keep a reasonable ratio of nitrogen to non-nitrogen energy in order to limit other complications (see Chapter 7).

Patients with severe renal impairment who are on dialysis or haemofiltration can often be given 'standard' IVN regimens since the dialysis can remove excess fluid and electrolytes. However, extreme care is needed to ensure that the IVN regimen is reviewed and usually changed when the dialysis is stopped.

Liver disease

Patients with liver disease often have considerable derangement in fluid and electrolyte regulation as well as deranged intake, processing and storage of both macronutrients and micronutrients. The provision of the correct feeding regimen can therefore be extremely challenging and indeed exactly what is required is open to debate. The provision of IVN can also cause liver problems, but these are discussed in Chapter 12.

- *Sodium and fluid*: patients with liver disease tend to be vasodilated and the low peripheral resistance results in a low blood pressure and hence poor renal perfusion. This in turn reduces salt and water clearance and triggers the renin-angiotensin system. The activation of that pathway results in high levels of aldosterone production and these, along with the fact that the metabolic clearance of aldosterone is often reduced (since it takes place in the liver), can lead to very high circulating aldosterone levels. These combine with the poor renal function to cause severe salt and water overload, often with clinical ascites and oedema.

Although plasma levels of sodium are often low in patients with liver disease, provision of sodium should normally be restricted to 40 mmol or less per day. This is because the low plasma sodium usually occurs in the context of raised with total body sodiums coupled with fluid retention that is even more dramatic. The sodium restriction must therefore be instigated with concurrent fluid restriction and, in most cases, liver patients with signs of fluid overload should receive only 1–2 litres in total from all fluid sources. Most are also put on diuretics to promote further salt and water clearance – especially spironolactone, which is an aldosterone antagonist. However, the restriction of both sodium and water sometimes needs to be avoided, especially with the development of worsening renal failure in the context of a low circulating volume. The development of severe, symptomatic hyponatraemia may also force a relaxation of sodium restriction.

In view of the above, management of sodium and fluid provision along with the use of concurrent diuretics is extremely difficult in liver patients and the key role for most IVN prescribers must be liaison with expert ward clinicians to ensure that overall aims for sodium and fluid restriction or provision are met.

- *Other electrolytes*: It is not unusual for the abnormalities in renal perfusion seen in liver patients to cause significant renal failure (hepatorenal syndrome) and under these circumstances all the prescribing considerations outlined for renal impairment (see above) will need to be followed.

- *Energy*: 'standard' levels of total energy provision are usually appropriate, taking into account the dangers of refeeding syndromes or overfeeding of very sick patients, as discussed in Chapters 8 and 9. The normal ratio of approximately 50% lipid to 50% carbohydrate for the non-protein energy supply is also suitable for most patients since the commonly met belief that a damaged liver is poor at metabolising lipid is not usually true.

- *Protein*: in general the traditional measure of restricting protein provision to liver patients should be avoided and 'standard' levels should be provided. However, we would recommend more limited early provision during the initial phase of feeding in sick patients for the same reasons as those outlined in Chapter 7 for all patient groups. Although restricting levels of protein provision can improve cerebral function in some patients with encephalopathy,

encephalopathy *per se* rarely contributes to the deterioration or death of liver patients, whereas restricting protein provision for prolonged periods could do so. Furthermore, studies of encephalopathic patients demonstrate better outcomes in those receiving more protein[1,2]. Studies in patients with chronic stable liver disease (i.e. cirrhosis without acute illness or injury) suggest that this group probably requires higher than normal levels of protein provision to come into nitrogen balance[3]. It therefore seems sensible to feed them at levels towards the upper end of recommended nitrogen provision once there are no contraindications for doing so. Many patients with liver disease have a low albumin, which may also contribute (to a small degree) to the development of ascites and fluid overload. However, the provision of IVN *per se* does not influence albumin in any patient group and hence low albumin in liver patients or others is not an indication for IVN support (see Chapter 3).

- *Micronutrients*: interpretation of plasma vitamin levels in patients with liver disease is difficult, e.g. reduced hepatic production of retinol-binding protein may suggest low vitamin A status when it is in fact normal. Nevertheless, many patients are likely to be depleted in several micronutrients and hence balanced provision, with twice normal levels during early feeding (see Chapter 9), would seem to be appropriate. Patients with alcoholic liver disease are particularly likely to be depleted in folate and vitamin C along with B-group vitamins, especially thiamine. It is absolutely essential that appropriate thiamine replacement is given before commencing feeding, e.g. using intravenous Pabrinex, to avoid precipitating Wernicke-Korsakoff syndrome (see Chapter 9).

Pancreatitis, pancreatic insufficiency and diabetes

The pancreas can be damaged by many different processes and it is not unusual for patients with pancreatic disease to require IVN. In the past, intravenous feeding was used routinely in the management of acute or acute-on-chronic pancreatitis, in the belief that limiting administration of any oral or enteral feed would limit stimulation of pancreatic digestive enzyme production and hence reduce autodigestive damage to the gland. In recent years, however, a number of studies comparing clinical outcomes with enteral feeding versus IVN in acute pancreatitis have demonstrated that enteral feeding is better[4-6]. It has been suggested that this is due to better maintenance of gut barrier function when enteral feed is present in the lumen but it could also be due to the fact that enteral feeding tends to have limited success whenever the pancreatitis is severe, because severe disease usually causes significant ileus. The IVN-fed groups in the studies that demonstrated the apparent superiority of the enteral route therefore received higher levels of feeding, which may have had disadvantages (see Chapter 7). Indeed, feeding by the enteral route does not grant benefit when compared to IVN feeding at levels low enough not to cause significant hyperglycaemia. Nevertheless, the studies do show that routine use of IVN is *not* indicated and the use of intravenous feeding in pancreatic disease should therefore be restricted to patients with complications causing intestinal failure or patients with vulnerable upper gastrointestinal anastomoses following surgical intervention.

Pancreatic exocrine functions are important in determining a patient's ability to digest oral or enteral feed and as such their failure may contribute to the need for IVN support. However, pancreatic exocrine failure *per se* does not alter the requirements for an IVN regimen. Pancreatic endocrine failure, on the other hand, leads to insufficient insulin production and hence can cause high glucose levels in patients on standard IVN. This can be dangerous and so many patients with pancreatic disease will require insulin on a sliding scale. Usually it is neither necessary nor appropriate to change the IVN regimen to gain control and patients should therefore be prescribed protein, carbohydrate and lipids at standard levels for their needs.

Insulin infusions will also be needed in most type 1 and type 2 diabetic patients requiring IVN and it is not unusual for acutely unwell patients to develop temporary insulin resistance that gives them a reversible form of the type 2 problem. Once again it is usually appropriate to start with the standard balance of macronutients within any IVN required, using insulin as necessary to control glucose levels. Blood glucose consistently above 11 mmol/L (or less in ITU settings) indicates the need for insulin but its incorporation within IVN bags is not recommended (see Appendix 1). In addition to hyperglycaemia, it is not unusual to see poor lipid clearance in type 2 diabetics and those with the stress-induced insulin resistance. Persistently lipaemic blood samples should trigger a reduction of the lipid component in your IVN regimen.

Cardiac failure

Cardiac function is dependent on plasma electrolyte levels. Great care must be taken when prescribing electrolytes in IVN regimens for patients with cardiac failure, especially as many patients will have 'hidden' electrolyte abnormalities on referral and many electrolyte abnormalities can result (see Chapter 8), along with the various potential electrolyte complications, from the use of IVN (see Chapter 12). Additionally, the fluid volume that the heart receives from the venous system (the preload) can influence cardiac function and so you must also be careful when prescribing the volume of the IVN regimen. While you should aim to maintain plasma electrolytes appropriately, it is worth giving specific consideration to:

- *Sodium and fluid*: a daily restriction of one or both may be in place. The sodium content can contribute to fluid retention and increase the cardiac preload, potentially worsening cardiac failure. You will need to ask one of the ward clinicians and if necessary modify your prescribing as required for the patient, but do consider whether other modifications to the patient may make your prescribing simpler (e.g. reducing supplemental infusions).
- *Potassium*: the ward clinicians may be aiming for a plasma potassium towards the upper end of the local laboratory reference range. You should clearly take this into account but very clear lines of communication are needed regarding the potassium in the IVN and how much is running concurrently (e.g. in separate infusions). Note that if supplemental potassium must be given due to inadequate IVN content, it will also provide a fluid load to the patient that may be undesirable (above).
- *Prescribed drugs* that may also influence fluid or electrolytes. For example, diuretics affect fluid and electrolyte losses that must be taken into account when prescribing.
- *Concurrent renal compromise* is often present and will complicate the picture because all considerations for renal impairment must then be considered (see above).

Respiratory failure

Lung function is driven by the level of carbon dioxide in the blood and can be compromised by overfeeding of glucose and/or lipid. You should normally prescribe as close to a 50:50 ratio of glucose and lipid as possible (see Chapter 7), but some patients may have a specific need for a different ratio (e.g. about 70:30 either way). This is not always necessary in patients with respiratory failure but does require consideration in conjunction with the ward clinicians for each individual case.

The metabolism of glucose increases carbon dioxide production because its respiratory quotient (RQ: the ratio of carbon dioxide produced by glucose metabolism versus the quantity of oxygen consumed) is 1.0. This compares to an RQ of 0.7 for the metabolism of lipid. Excess provision of glucose may therefore increase problems for patients with respiratory failure dominated by carbon dioxide retention whereas excess provision of lipid energy will increase problems in hypoxic respiratory failure.

Short-bowel syndrome and high-output gastrointestinal fistulae

SBS is a condition of partial or complete intestinal failure caused by inadequate functional length of one or more critical regions of the gastrointestinal tract[7]. It is most commonly seen as a consequence of extensive surgical resection or resections of the jejunum and/or ileum and/or colon as a consequence of superior mesenteric infarction or Crohn's disease. However, it can also occur after surgical interventions for a wide variety of intra-abdominal pathologies, including invasive malignancy, sclerosing damage from radiotherapy and even recurrent complications and anastomotic breakdowns from non-gastrointestinal surgical intervention. In addition, fistulae to the skin from high in the small intestine can result in a physiological/nutritional state that needs to be managed in much the same way as SBS.

Patients with SBS or high-output fistulae often need IVN, especially in the early weeks after surgery. Frequently, the patients have jejunal or ileal stomas but later they may be rejoined, if functional colon remains, so that they have jejunocolic or ileocolic anastomoses. The specific nutritional and IVN-related problems of SBS patients depend largely on their remaining length of jejunum and ileum and whether that remainder is healthy. Difficulties arise from not only inadequate absorption of macronutrients, micronutrients, electrolytes and fluids but also their excessive losses via the stoma or fistula. Rejoining of the colon can markedly improve losses, particularly of electrolytes and fluid.

Most new SBS/fistulae patients are initially nil by mouth following their last surgical resection and, since re-establishment of adequate oral or enteral feeding will almost certainly be very delayed and may be unachievable, IVN should be established as soon as possible. This should then be continued while the patient recovers from surgery and the absorptive capacity of the remaining gut is assessed. This will tend to improve slowly with time and the correction of any nutritional, fluid or electrolyte deficits. No final decision that a patient is unable to become independent of IVN or intravenous fluids should therefore be made until the patient is repleted and all metabolic stresses of surgery have settled. Even then, with more time patients may show adaptations that will improve their limited gastrointestinal function, especially if they have remaining ileum or can have any colon rejoined (see below).

SBS patients and those with high fistulae are best characterised within anatomical groups.

Jejunostomy patients and patients with high jejunal fistulae

Carbohydrate, protein and many vitamins are normally absorbed in the jejunum and reduction of effective jejunal length can cause protein/energy malnutrition and multiple vitamin deficiencies. In addition, oral foods and drinks are multiplied in volume three- to fourfold by saliva, gastric, biliary and upper intestinal secretions. This results in large volumes of salty fluid (about 90 mmol/L) entering the upper jejunum and, if this is then lost via a stoma or fistula, the patients become very prone to salt and water depletion. To make matters worse, the more the patients eat and drink, the more fluid may be lost. They also tend to suffer from magnesium, calcium and vitamin deficiencies.

If a patient has < 100 cm of remaining healthy jejunum, long-term IVN support, either daily or intermittently, will usually be required and the need for IVN support is almost invariable with < 50 cm. Patients with > 100 cm of jejunum can often be maintained in fluid balance using aggressive oral salt replacement, while limiting hypotonic fluids whereas those with a jejunum < 100 cm and a stoma usually remain net secretors of salt and water. They therefore need intravenous or subcutaneous fluid and sodium supplementation, even if they can absorb enough macro-nutrients to avoid the need for full IVN.

Reintroduction of fluids and food by the oral/enteral route should be stepwise and slower than would normally be the case following gastrointestinal surgery. This permits time for the re-establishment of gut motility and regeneration of gut mucosa. Introduction of fluids should precede the introduction of oral nutrients in the conventional pattern, i.e. sips, 30 mL/hour, 60 mL/hour, free fluids (see Figure 4.3 in Chapter 4). Water should be used initially, introducing nutritious drinks once patients are able to tolerate 60 mL/hour. Readily absorbable polymeric preparations can be used with advice from dietitians. Elemental diets with high osmolality will make things worse rather than better since they cause osmotic movement of even more water into the gut lumen and hence promote increased stomal/fistula losses. The early introduction of small quantities of liquid nutrition will help to promote mucosal regeneration but you should avoid exceeding the current absorptive capacity of the gut (manifest by large increases in stomal losses), since this will grant no advantage and will simply make attainment of nutrient and fluid balance more difficult. It is better to cut back, waiting for further adaptive changes and trying measures to improve the situation. These measures include:

- *Salt supplementation of liquids*: losses of salt and water are decreased by the addition of salt to oral/enteral fluids to give concentrations of > 90 mmol/L and ideally around 100–120 mmol/L[8]. Salty drinks (which may be suitably flavoured) can be obtained from pharmacy and served chilled. Potential formulations, including suggestions on how to increase the sodium content of standard oral supplements/enteral feeds, are shown in Appendix 4. Most patients gain benefit if they consume up to about 1 L/day of these high-salt (St Marks) fluids, but few gain by consuming more. If the jejunum is very short, patients will remain net secretors anyway and, if that is the case, it seems unnecessary to make them consume an unpleasant drink when IVN or intravenous fluids are to be given regularly and adequate sodium and water status can be maintained via that route. Some patients will not drink the salty fluid but can benefit by receiving it via an enteral tube. If they then require long-term gastrointestinal salt supplementation, a gastrostomy may be valuable.
- *Restriction of non-salt-containing, hypotonic fluids*: this usually needs to be limited to 1–1.5 litres in the long run but early after surgery it may be necessary to continue avoiding all oral/enteral intake even beyond any normal postoperative concerns about ileus or anastamoses. This is to minimise stomal or fistula losses whilst regaining metabolic balance and control. When the patient is more stable, you can allow a slow increase in oral hypotonic fluid intake while strictly monitoring stool losses, fluid balance and serum and urinary sodium levels. This will allow you to determine the individual patient's daily current limit for oral hypotonic fluid. Ensure that the patient understands why oral hypotonic fluid intake increases losses and why drinking small quantities frequently might

limit total output compared to drinking similar overall volumes but in larger amounts less frequently.

- *Antimotility drugs*: drugs such as loperamide and codeine phosphate, in high dose, either alone or in combination, are best given 30 minutes before meals. An attempt to assess their benefits should be made since they are often of little value in reducing jejunostomy output.
- *Octreotide* may be useful in reducing liquid losses in high-output jejunal stomas. However, it is unlikely that net secretors can be changed to net absorbers. Overall, it is probably worth trying for 2–3 days with pre- and post-commencement monitoring of stomal outputs to see if any benefit has accrued.
- *24-hour use of the limited absorptive capacity*: consider overnight slow feeding via nasogastric tube or, if longer-term, via a percutaneous gastrostomy (PEG) in order to maximise nutritional status without the need for IVN. Sip-feeds, with salt supplementation if necessary, should be encouraged between meals and the enteral feeds can also be salt-supplemented (see Appendix 4).
- Magnesium and calcium deficiencies are likely in jejunostomy patients and oral or IVN supplementation may be required. 1-alpha-hydroxy-vitamin D_3 can help with both deficiencies in doses of 1–3 µg/day.

IVN for jejunostomy patients and patients with high-output fistulae will almost certainly need to be high-volume (4 L/day is commonly needed) and usually requires very high sodium levels, with some patients on 300–400 mmol/day. In some cases, bag size and stability issues necessitate additional separate normal saline infusions. Close monitoring of hydration, salt and electrolyte status is required, initially on a daily basis. This should include daily fluid balance, body weight, lying and standing blood pressure, urea, creatinine and electrolytes. Most importantly, net sodium status is best assessed through random urine tests that may contain very low (often < 10 mmol/L) sodium levels in depleted patients. Magnesium and calcium requirements may also be very high and urinary potassium losses can be a problem because of secondary hyperaldosteronism (triggered by the body's sodium and fluid depletion) and the fact that magnesium depletion also leads to poor renal retention of potassium.

Once reasonable quantities of liquid feeds are absorbed, solid diets should be started slowly. If patients have a colonic mucous fistula likely to be rejoined in the future, it is advantageous to put small quantities of the jejunostomy output into the colonic fistula on a daily basis. This will help to maintain the health of the colon. Where appropriate, patients should be advised sooner rather than later that there may be a permanent need for IVN in order to commence home IVN training. This may shorten their hospital admission if home IVN is eventually required.

Jejunocolic anastomosis patients

A jejunocolic anastomosis provides additional capacity for the absorption of nutrients, especially carbohydrate, salt and water. Patients with more than 50 cm of jejunum anastomosed to the colon can often maintain macronutrient, salt and water balance without parenteral supplements, especially after the colon has had time to adapt. Patients with less than 50 cm of jejunum rejoined to the colon usually continue to need long-term IVN. Loss of the terminal ileum leads to poor reabsorption of bile salts and jejunocolic anastomoses patients often have bile-salt-induced diarrhoea.

IVN considerations for these patients are similar to those for patients with jejunal stomas, although less extreme sodium, water and electrolyte replacement is usually needed. All strategies applied to jejunostomy patients (see above) also need to be considered for these patients but the chances of achieving successful nutritional and fluid balance without intravenous supplementation are much enhanced. Colestyramine may help in bile-salt-induced diarrhoea but must be used with caution as it may deplete the bile salt pool and worsen both steatorrhoea and gallstone formation. Renal stones may form secondary to dehydration and oxalate reabsorption. Dietary avoidance of oxalate may be indicated.

Long-term adaptations in intestinal function may be considerable and hence periodic review of absorptive capacity is needed. Many rejoined patients initially requiring IVN do not need it in the long term.

Ileostomy and ileocolic anastomosis patients

Most patients who have lost ileum do not suffer from complete intestinal failure, although they may have poor fat absorption and are prone to specific deficiencies of the fat-soluble vitamins A, D, E and K. Vitamin B_{12} may also be low with terminal ileal resection. Salt and water balance is normally maintained without difficulty, although magnesium and calcium balance can be problematic. Some adaptation of ileal absorptive capacity can be expected, especially if the terminal ileum is preserved.

Patients with ileocolic anastomoses show even greater adaptation and most rejoined patients who initially require IVN will not need it in the long term.

Most steps and strategies applying to jejunostomy patients help with ileal resections, e.g. high-dose loperamide with or without codeine or dihydrocodeine, although most will not need high-salt drinks or tight restrictions on hypotonic fluids and, if IVN is required, its content can often be close to that used for standard patients.

References

1.   Morgan T, MoritzT, Mendenhall C, Haas R. Protein consumption and hepatic encephalopathy in alcoholic hepatitis. VA Cooperative Study Group #275. *J Am Coll Nutr* 1995; 14: 152–158.

2.   Soulsby C, Morgan M. Dietary management of hepatic encephalopathy in cirrhotic patients: survey of current practice in United Kingdom. *Br Med J* 1999; 318: 1391.

3.   Nielsen K, Kondrup J, Martinsen L *et al*. Nutritional assessment and adequacy of dietary intake in hospitalized patients with alcoholic liver cirrhosis. *Br J Nutr* 1993; 69: 665–679.

4.   McClave S, Greene L, Snider H *et al*. Comparison of the safety of early enteral vs parenteral nutrition in mild acute pancreatitis. *J Parenteral Enteral Nutr* 1997; 21: 14–20.

5.   Kalfarentzos F, Kehagais J, Mead N *et al*. Enteral nutrition is superior to parenteral nutrition in severe acute pancreatitis: results of a randomized prospective trial. *Br J Surg* 1997; 84: 1665–1669.

6.   Windsor A, Kanwar S, Barnes E *et al*. Compared with parenteral nutrition, enteral feeding attenuates the acute phase response and improves disease severity in acute pancreatitis. *Gut* 1998; 42: 431–435.

7.   Nightingale J. The short bowel. In: Nightingale J, ed. *Intestinal Failure*. London: Greenwich Medical Media, 2001: 177–200.

8.   Nightingale J, Lennard-Jones J, Walker E, Farthing M. Oral salt supplements for jejunostomy losses: comparison of sodium chloride capsules, glucose electrolyte solution, and glucose polymer electrolyte solution. *Gut* 1992; 33: 759–761.

11

Regimen choice

Introduction

The choice of intravenous nutrition (IVN) regimens that could be used in any individual patient is almost infinite and, frequently, more than one regimen may be suitable for the same clinical situation. Whatever your decision, the regimen must always be practical and safe. In this chapter, we discuss our approach to choosing regimens which, although based on the theoretical considerations already covered in this book, is often pragmatic rather than firmly evidence-based.

Your first decision is to select the macronutrient base of your prescription. This may be a precompounded and sterilised triple-chamber bag, a previously aseptically compounded bag or a regimen that you design entirely from basic components. Following this, you will need to prescribe additions to the basic bag to form a complete regimen which will always include micronutrients and usually electrolytes. There may also be other additions, including extra fluid or specialised components such as glutamine. Without exception, all additions to an IVN regimen must be carried out in a sterile environment within a Technical Services unit (see Chapter 15).

Precompounded and sterilised triple-chamber bags

Precompounded, sterilised triple-chamber bags are nearly always the simplest and most cost-effective option on which to base your prescription. They consist of three individual compartments which contain nitrogen, glucose and lipid. Dividing them are weak seals which can be broken when the bag is rolled up. The three separate components then mix yet retain a closed, sterile system (Figure 11.1).

These bags are extremely useful but do have some disadvantages (Table 11.1).

All commercial manufacturers of IVN components have a range of triple bags available, varying in the type of macronutrients included

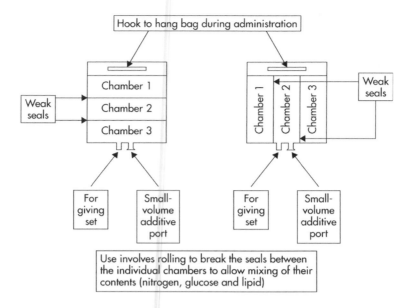

Figure 11.1 Precompounded and terminally sterilised triple-chamber macronutrient bags.

(e.g. the lipid), the energy provided by each macronutrient, the volume of the bag when mixed and stability limits for additions. Despite having some disadvantages (Table 11.1), it is likely that the advantages are sufficient to warrant their use for the majority of your patients. Nevertheless, you must never assume that just because they are commercially available, these bags are always appropriate for your patient. This needs to be assessed on an individual basis.

In some cases, the use of precompounded bags may be limited by the range that you stock locally. For example, you may have nothing appropriate for use in a patient with renal failure who is retaining electrolytes and/or fluid. When this occurs, you will need to consider whether you can use a proportion of a bag, running it over a longer duration, or, if absolutely necessary, whether you need to design an individualised regimen (see below).

Choosing a regimen

Once you have determined the full-rate macronutrient requirements of your patient, i.e. those that would be likely to meet current needs if that was your initial aim (see Chapter 7), you can select the regimen on

Table 11.1 Advantages and disadvantages of precompounded and sterilised triple-chamber intravenous nutrition bags

Advantages	Disadvantages
Licensed products approved by the Licensing Authority	Apparent 'ready-to-go' nature may tempt people to treat them as ward stock (never appropriate)
Large stocks available from the manufacturer	Macronutrient content in the range may be problematic (for example, minimum volume for a fluid-restricted patient)
Available in a range containing variable amounts of macronutrients	
Have long shelf-life, limiting wastage	Appearance during administration often not pharmaceutically elegant (the fluid pools at the bottom of the bag)
Can typically be stored at room temperature before use	
Reduce aseptic manipulation of macronutrients	Each will have a minimum electrolyte content that cannot be removed
Standardised stability data available from the manufacturer	Frequent requirement to 'top up' electrolyte content
Often resource-efficient (time and purchase cost) for macronutrients	The alcohol used to kill surface contamination in Technical Services (see Chapter 15) can cause peeling of the bag text
	Resource costs of many electrolyte additions can quickly add up (time and purchase cost)

which to base your IVN prescription. This often requires some compromise.

Your first decision is whether you have a suitable precompounded and sterilised triple chamber bag that closely matches your patient's energy and nitrogen needs. However, it is neither necessary nor possible for you to stock the entire range of available precompounded, sterilised triple-chamber bags due to problems of local storage, logistics and costs. Nutrition teams and Technical Services therefore make decisions on which regimens to stock routinely (see Chapter 15), sometimes giving the range of locally stocked bags clinically useful names such as 'low', 'medium' and 'high', matched to groups of patients with low, medium or high macronutrient requirements. This can make prescribing simpler (see below). Additional descriptive names such as 'low-volume electrolyte-free' and 'repletion' may also prove useful depending on the range of bags stocked.

Matching energy requirements

An exact match between your estimated daily energy requirements (see Chapter 7) and a stock bag is rarely possible, but you can usually find a bag within ±200 kcal. However, because of our concerns with over-feeding of sick patients (see Chapter 7), we prefer to avoid excess feeding of even 200 kcal and aim instead for limits of −200 to +100 kcal. We therefore round down towards −200 kcal if there is a choice, particu-larly in very-low-weight or very sick patients who are at high risk of refeeding electrolyte or micronutrient problems (see Chapters 8 and 9). You can, of course, prescribe a proportion of a regimen to limit energy, fluid or electrolyte provision although, if you do so, extra electrolyte additions are often needed in order to ensure correct provision (see below).

You may also need to underfeed significantly if you are using peripheral vein feeding (see Chapter 3), since reducing the risks of peripheral thrombophlebitis requires regimens of lower osmolality (see Chapter 7). For example, if you only stock bags with 1200 and 2200 kcal and your estimated requirements are 1800 kcal, you will have to choose the lower option until more suitable intravenous access is secured and the patient is nutritionally stable.

Matching nitrogen requirements

If the macronutrient bags that you keep have been carefully selected to provide an appropriate ratio of non-nitrogen energy to grams of nitrogen (see Chapter 7), it is likely that matching the energy in the bag to the patient's requirement will also provide an appropriate quantity of nitrogen. However, if your patient has very specific nitrogen require-ments he or she may require a different regimen, although this is unlikely, particularly in the initial stages of refeeding.

Electrolyte additions

Changes in the electrolyte content of precompounded bags should only be made if clinically relevant in order to prevent unnecessary Technical Services workload and other staff basing their management decisions on changes that are unlikely to be relevant. The additions must also be stable and many electrolyte products not only modify a single electrolyte level but actually alter two or even more, depending on the salt used (see Chapter 8 and Appendix 2). Examples of products that you may

Table 11.2 Hypothetical regimens for the example given in the text

Regimen	Nitrogen (g)	Energy (kcal)	Volume (mL)		Na	K	Mg	Ca	PO₄
					Electrolyte content in total bag (mmol)				
A*	6	1200	1500	Minimum	40	30	2	2	10
				Maximum	175	200	6	6	18
B*	10	1500	2000	Minimum	64	48	3.2	3.2	16
				Maximum	295	300	10	10	30

Na, sodium; K, potassium; Mg, magnesium; Ca, calcium; PO₄, phosphate.
* Both regimens would also require the addition of vitamins and trace elements (see Chapter 9).

stock are shown in Appendix 2 and you should ensure that you have a sufficient range to meet likely local requirements.

Table 11.2 illustrates the practical inclusion of electrolytes into a macronutrient bag. Two hypothetical regimens are shown along with the hypothetical stability restrictions on total electrolyte content.

Based on these hypothetical regimens, various rates of administration are considered to illustrate restrictions when prescribing 'standard' daily requirements in IVN regimens (see Chapter 8). The values would need to be modified if the patient had specific electrolyte requirements (see Chapters 8 and 10):

- *Regimen A at quarter-rate of 16 mL/hour:*
    - Sodium 40 mmol plus any from the phosphate source
    - Potassium 240 mmol to give 60 mmol/day – exceeds stability but total of sodium and potassium is below the combined limit
    - Magnesium 6 mmol limited by stability
    - Calcium 6 mmol limited by stability
    - Phosphate 18 mmol limited by stability

- *Regimen A at half-rate of 32 mL/hour:*
    - Sodium 40 mmol plus any from the phosphate source
    - Potassium 120 mmol to give 60 mmol/day
    - Magnesium 6 mmol limited by stability
    - Calcium 6 mmol limited by stability
    - Phosphate 18 mmol limited by stability

- *Regimen A at full-rate of 63 mL/hour:*
  - Sodium 40 mmol plus any from the phosphate source
  - Potassium 60 mmol
  - Magnesium 5 mmol
  - Calcium 5 mmol
  - Phosphate 18 mmol limited by stability

- *Regimen B at quarter-rate of 21 mL/hour:*
  - Sodium 64 mmol plus any from the phosphate source
  - Potassium 240 mmol to give 60 mmol/day
  - Magnesium 10 mmol limited by stability
  - Calcium 10 mmol limited by stability
  - Phosphate 30 mmol limited by stability

- *Regimen B at half-rate of 42 mL/hour:*
  - Sodium 64 mmol plus any from the phosphate source
  - Potassium 120 mmol to give 60 mmol/day
  - Magnesium 10 mmol
  - Calcium 10 mmol
  - Phosphate 30 mmol limited by stability

- *Regimen B at full-rate of 83 mL/hour:*
  - Sodium 64 mmol plus any from the phosphate source
  - Potassium 60 mmol
  - Magnesium 5 mmol
  - Calcium 5 mmol
  - Phosphate 25 mmol

Note that the use of a lower-energy bag at half-rate instead of a higher energy bag at quarter-rate would limit the need for so much potassium in the bag (risk management consideration) and would probably allow relatively more calcium, magnesium and phosphate to be included.

The need to make judgements on whether any electrolyte additions are really of clinical importance is covered in Chapters 8 and 10. If prescribing on a mmol/kg basis, consider the total quantity prescribed in context. For example, 1 mmol/kg potassium for a 70-kg patient would mean a total of 70 mmol. If there was already 67 mmol in the bag, the addition is insignificant because 67 mmol/70 kg = 0.96 mmol/kg, which easily rounds to 1 mmol/kg.

Ward electrolyte prescribing

There may be circumstances when your prescription falls short of covering estimated requirements because of additional action that is to be taken on the wards. A common example is for patients who are hypokalaemic, for whom potassium infusions are planned independently of the potassium supplied in your IVN. When this is the case you must ensure that the additional actions are actually carried out (especially if the patient is moving wards) and that those responsible for the additional actions are aware of, and accounting for, the content of the IVN that your patient will receive. See also Chapter 6.

Compromising on electrolyte additions due to stability (most likely with magnesium, calcium and phosphate) may also require additional, separate electrolyte supplementation (see Chapters 8 and 12).

Micronutrient additions

Every prescription that you write must include micronutrients and so-called emergency IVN is never an indication for not making the necessary additions (see Chapter 16). You will always need to stock appropriate vitamins and trace elements. We recommend the routine provision of double vitamins, while limiting iron, during the initial 10–14 days of IVN followed by maintenance micronutrient provision with iron (see Chapter 9). You must always confirm stability for any micronutrient additions.

Other additions

Specialist additions to IVN regimens such as additional fluid or glutamine may be required locally and all should be confirmed as stable in your chosen regimen before prescribing (see Appendix 1).

Approximation of regimen volume

The macronutrient bag that you have selected will always require micronutrient additions and often the addition of fluids and electrolytes. Every addition will increase the volume of the bag. Many Technical Services units (see Chapter 15) have specialised compounding software that can calculate the theoretical final volume of the bag. However, if using paper prescriptions and worksheets (see below), it is helpful to approximate the final bag volume to the nearest 100 mL, using

Table 11.3 Examples of approximating intravenous nutrition (IVN) macronutrient bag volume

	Bag volume (mL)	Full-rate* (mL/hour per 24 hours)	Half-rate* (mL/hour per 24 hours)	Quarter-rate* (mL/hour per 24 hours)
Nominal IVN bag volume	1420	59	30	15
(mL)	1810	75	38	19
	2070	86	43	22
Nominal IVN bag volume	1500	63	32	16
after small-volume additions	1890	79	40	20
(mL) (80 mL per bag in this	2150	90	45	23
example table)				
Approximation of bag volume	1400	58	29	15
(mL)	1800	75	38	19
	2100	88	44	22
Error of approximation	1400	−8%	−5%	−2%
compared to actual volume	1800	−5%	−3%	−1%
after additions (based on 24	2100	−2%	−1%	−1%
hour infusion volume)				

* See Chapter 7 for an explanation of full-rate, half-rate and quarter rate.

theoretical pre-addition volumes (Table 11.3). This will inevitably introduce some variation into your prescribing, although the bags are typically overfilled by 4–5% (and possibly by as much as 10% if you are designing your own regimen). Therefore your rate approximation will go some way to limiting the error of the nominal bag volume.

Designing your own regimen

Designing your own regimen is time-consuming for both you and Technical Services. It also tends to be more expensive, especially if particular components need to be ordered in. Before going down this road, you should therefore exhaust any other options for using precompounded, sterilised triple-chamber bags, including giving only a proportion of the bag or running the bag over a longer duration (subject to stability constraints). Nevertheless, although most hospitals only use their own regimens for patients with very unusual needs, some find that the needs of their own local nutrition service are better met by designing a range of local 'standard' regimens than by using precompounded

Table 11.4 Advantages and disadvantages of specially designed intravenous nutrition bags to be aseptically compounded for routine local use

Advantages	Disadvantages
Promotes relationships with the supplying company	Unlicensed product
Bags are made to your precise specification (you may find that a particular balance of macronutrients suits the majority of your patients)	Compounding difficulties may limit availability (you will need a contingency plan)
	Logistics may be complex or restrictive; must have a validated 'cold chain' (see Appendix 1)
Allows you to specify electrolyte content with more realistic levels than most triple-chamber bags	Each bag will have a minimum electrolyte content that cannot be removed
May be able to vary bag content, e.g. electrolytes, by changing order	Storage in a refrigerator only (see Appendix 1) with a relatively short shelf-life
Bags usually more pharmaceutically elegant than precompounded and sterilised triple-chamber bags	Bags are compounded aseptically and not terminally sterilised, so risk of contamination is higher than with triple-chamber bags (however, actual risk is likely to be very low)
Reduces in-house aseptic manipulation of macronutrients for specialist regimens often used locally, saving time	
May allow pre-added micronutrients, reducing the need for routine additions by Technical Services	Pre-added micronutrients have significant cost and likely very short expiry; unlikely to be practical
The manufacturer may offer specific stability data and/or testing if you buy in sufficient quantity	May still require electrolyte additions (time and purchase cost)
Often resource-efficient (time and purchase cost) for macronutrients	Cost likely to be high (but required electrolyte additions may be considerably lower)

triple-chamber bags. This approach has both advantages and disadvantages (Table 11.4).

In most units, precompounded and sterilised triple-chamber bags are used unless an individual patient has special requirements. The most likely indications for designing your own regimen are therefore the need for:

- Fluid restriction
- Electrolyte restriction
- Unusual macronutrient ratios

- Alternative lipid type
- Lipid-free IVN

When there is no choice but to design your own regimen, you will need to take the following steps:

1. Determine the requirements for the IVN regimen (volume, nitrogen, glucose, lipid, electrolytes and micronutrients).
2. Accept that some compromise may be necessary and check with Technical Services (see Chapter 15) whether part containers of macronutrients may be used.
3. Begin by selecting a nitrogen source. These are typically available with or without electrolytes but, where possible, use one that contains electrolytes in order to limit subsequent electrolyte additions. If designing a very-low-volume bag, it is likely you will require a highly concentrated nitrogen source of around 20 g/L. Otherwise it is usual to select a source providing the approximate quantity of nitrogen that your patient requires in grams per 1000 mL of product (if available).
4. Select a lipid source, if required, usually aiming to provide 40–50% of the non-nitrogen energy from lipid (see Chapter 7).
5. Use glucose to make up to the required volume, selecting strength(s) that will achieve the total required energy whilst giving an appropriate final volume (see below and Appendix 2).
6. Add electrolytes if required, with phosphate first, since increasing the phosphate will also increase one or more other electrolytes (see Chapter 8 and Appendix 2).
7. Add the required vitamins and trace elements.
8. Double-check your calculations.
9. Assess the stability of the potential IVN regimen.
10. If necessary, consider whether it is suitable for peripheral administration (see Chapters 3 and 7).

These steps are most easily carried out in the form of a table (Figure 11.2).

Stability issues

IVN component manufacturers provide generic standard stability tables for compounding individual regimens which allow creativity but require accurate interpretation to be useful. Always double-check whether values given are per bag or per litre.

Adult intravenous nutrition formula calculation

Patient: _____ Ward: _____ Date: _____ Item number: _____

Nutritional parameter	Ingredient	Volume (mL)	Weight (g)	Protein (g of N)	Nitrogen (kcal)	Glucose (kcal)	Lipid (kcal)	Total energy (kcal)	Na (mmol)	K (mmol)	Mg (mmol)	Ca (mmol)	PO$_4$ (mmol)	Cl (mmol)	Zn (μmol)	Se (μmol)	Vits (mL)
	Prescription																
Protein																	
Lipid																	
Glucose																	
Electrolytes																	
Trace elements, vitamins and others																	
	Total																

Notes

Calculated by _____ Checked by _____ Stability _____

Figure 11.2 Table to assist in designing intravenous nutrition regimens.

On some occasions you may need to compound a regimen not covered by these tables. If this is the case then you will need to confirm stability directly with the relevant manufacturer by telephoning its support line. Written confirmation that the regimen is stable (e.g. a fax) will be needed before releasing the compounded regimen from Technical Services (see Chapter 15) and hence it is important to design a regimen that is likely to be stable before discussing it with the manufacturer. This will save both you and the manufacturer time. The stability of any regimen you have designed may be limited to 7 days regardless of whether the theoretical stability is longer due to licensing regulations (see Chapter 15). The addition of vitamins and trace elements usually limits stability to a maximum of 14 days due to the rapid breakdown of some of these additions (see Appendix 1).

Guidance on the general mixing of nitrogen sources and the use of glucose ranges in stability tables is given below.

Nitrogen and stability

Nitrogen is available in a number of forms from each commercial manufacturer and tends to enhance the stability of IVN regimens (see Appendix 1). For this reason, when you need to mix nitrogen products to achieve a different overall concentration (e.g. using 500 mL 9 g nitrogen per litre plus 500 mL 14 g nitrogen per litre is equivalent to using 1000 mL of 11.5 g nitrogen per litre), you should use the stability data for the *lower* level of nitrogen. Remember that you must only mix nitrogen sources that are the same in all respects other than the quantity of nitrogen per unit volume. Do not mix different manufacturers' products and do not mix different types of product from the same manufacturer.

Glucose and stability

The standard stability tables often include ranges. For example, they may state 1500–2500 mL of 10–30% w/v glucose. Under these circumstances, you are not necessarily restricted to using the specified glucose concentrations as long as the *overall* glucose volume and concentration are *equivalent* to that within the range specified in the standard stability data (Box 11.1).

Stability considerations of other components

The stability of IVN regimens is considered in Appendix 1, including various other components of IVN regimens.

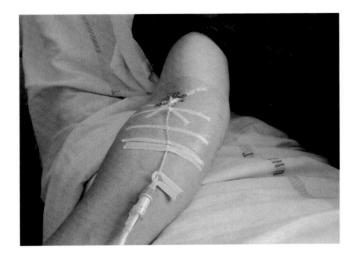

Plate 1 Midlines reduce IVN risks compared to using a central line as well as being less likely to result in peripheral vein thrombophlebitis compared to using a peripheral cannula.

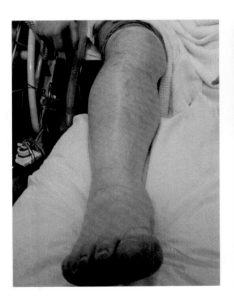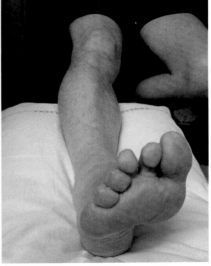

Plates 2a and 2b It is always helpful to examine patients for peripheral oedema which can mask evidence of wasting as well as to monitor for resolution of the oedema.

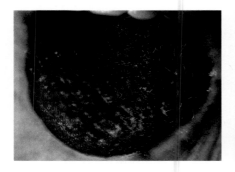

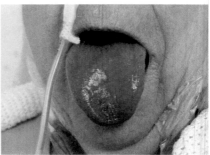

Plate 3a Red and rough ('raw steak') tongue suggestive of B vitamin deficiency.

Plate 3b Pale and smooth tongue suggestive of iron deficiency.

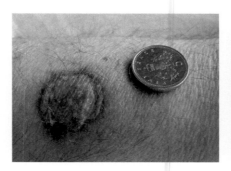

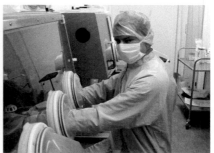

Plate 4 Subcutaneous extravasation and subsequent tissue necrosis can result from the use IVN, a particular risk when a peripheral cannula is used.

Plate 5 All IVN regimens are compounded in Technical Services within a dedicated cabinet. The environment and operator clothing are designed to minimise background contamination to limit the risk to the product during compounding.

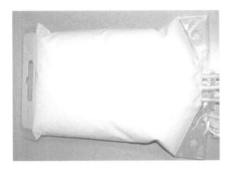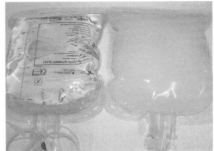

Plates 6a and 6b It is important to recognise the usual appearance of lipid regimens (a) and lipid free regimens (b, left) to help identify compounding errors (b, right).

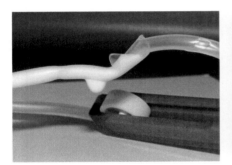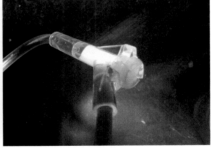

Plates 7a and 7b Always inspect bags and giving sets for damage which may be obvious (tear in a) or more difficult to detect (crack in b).

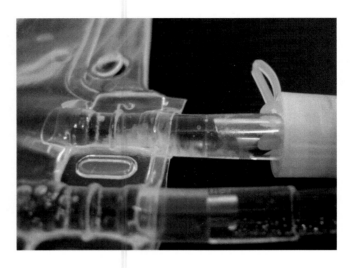

Plate 8 Regimen stability must always be considered and limits maximum component content of a regimen. It also requires adding components in the correct order to prevent local precipitation by the additive port.

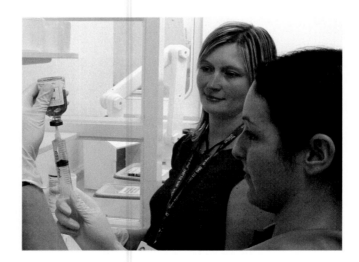

Plate 9 Regular validation of operators using manipulations of growth medium is important to ensure accurate aseptic technique when compounding products for patients.

Box 11.1 Equivalents to 1500–2500 mL of 10–30% w/v glucose

Examples

2000 mL of 10% w/v glucose or

500 mL 5% w/v glucose and 1000 mL 20% w/v glucose (overall 15% w/v) or

500 mL 5% w/v glucose and 1500 mL 20% w/v glucose (overall 16.3% w/v) or

1000 mL of 50% w/v glucose and 1000 mL water for injection (overall 25% w/v)

See Appendix 2 for how to carry out the necessary calculations

Macronutrient components for individualised IVN regimens

An adequate range of macronutrient ingredients is needed for local compounding to meet the specific requirements of individual patients. When deciding which components to stock you need to consider several factors, including:

- *Existing IVN contracts*: you will probably be obliged to keep products from the company that you are contracted to. However, you can usually use the products of a competing company when necessary, although this should be the exception and you may need to pay a premium for purchasing off-contract.
- *Frequency of ordering and delivery*: this will affect how quickly you can respond to the specific needs of an individual patient if you do not keep the required products in stock.
- *Range of precompounded macronutrient bags stocked*: if you do not stock particular bags, such as a low-volume, low-electrolyte regimen, you will need to be prepared to make individualised bags more often or have arrangements in place to obtain more specialised precompounded products quickly.
- *Flexibility of stocked products*: you need to be able to respond to a range of situations swiftly and this will influence your stock. Keeping a high-concentration nitrogen source, for example, enables low-volume bags to be compounded more easily.
- *Storage space*: room for stores and whether products need to be refrigerated will clearly influence your choices.
- *Number of IVN patients*: fewer patients means more risk of wasting expired stock of more specialist components.

- *Cost*: funds tied up in shelf stock may need to be limited depending on turnover (see above).

Since it is impossible to plan for every eventuality, there will be occasions when you must compromise on the regimen that you prescribe based on availability and practicality.

Regimen compromise

If you do not have or cannot individually compound the regimen that you require, or you are unable to make the electrolyte additions that you would ideally prescribe, you will need to consider whether you can make a clinically acceptable prescribing compromise:

- *Is another regimen choice clinically acceptable?* If necessary, always prescribe less energy and nitrogen rather than more, except for stable patients on long-term IVN to whom giving more may be reasonable. You may also be able to administer a proportion of a regimen but you must still ensure an appropriate electrolyte content for each 24-hour period. The use of peripheral intravenous access for IVN administration may require a significant compromise on energy and nitrogen provision (see Chapter 12).
- *Can a tailor-made regimen be compounded?* This is less desirable than modifying a precompounded macronutrient regimen due to the additional work, risk and cost. It may be appropriate in some circumstances (see above).
- *Can the prescription still include appropriate and adequate micronutrients?* It is essential that the micronutrient content at least provides the patient's basic needs. More specialised micronutrient additions (see Chapter 9) can be excluded for a limited time period if absolutely necessary and you may be able to consider the administration of Pabrinex separately to the IVN infusion. Note that some patients have a specific requirement for certain micronutrients that must always be met (see Chapter 9).
- *Can the prescribed electrolyte levels be amended with adjustments on the ward to allow the regimen to be used?* The ward may be able to cut back on existing electrolyte infusions or to prescribe further infusions as appropriate. Note that further electrolyte infusions come with a fluid load that may be unacceptable (see Chapter 7) and also require additional intravenous access, which may not be available or an increase in the risk of line sepsis due to additional manipulations. Fluid infusions with or without

electrolytes must be supported by specific stability data if concurrently run through the same lumen as the IVN (see Appendix 1).

- *Should I prescribe a regimen that may be inappropriate?* No. You will be responsible for your prescribing decisions and although you must be prepared to be practical, you must never prescribe anything that could realistically compromise the care of your patient.

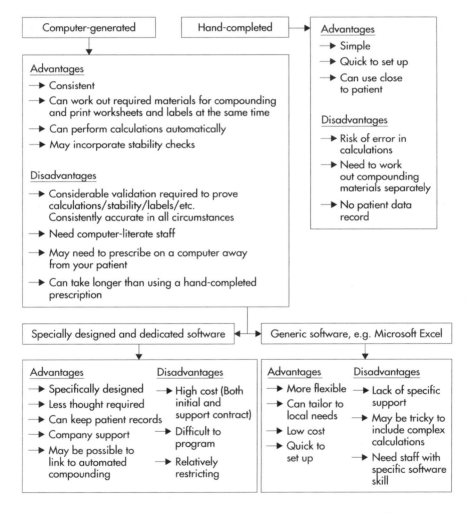

Figure 11.3 Choosing between hand-written and computer-generated intravenous nutrition prescription charts.

Table 11.5 Choice of documentation for writing intravenous nutrition (IVN) prescriptions

Option	Advantages	Disadvantages
Medicine chart	Readily read by other staff. Constant reminder that your patient is prescribed IVN	May not be sufficient room for detail of IVN contents. Chart may be off the ward when you need to prescribe further IVN. The chart would need to be off the ward for compounding and release*
Specifically designed and dedicated space on medicine chart	Readily read by other staff. Constant reminder that your patient is prescribed IVN. Should be sufficient space for IVN prescription detail	Need for the dedicated IVN section would be uncommon and so space could be more effectively used. Chart may be off the ward when you need to prescribe further IVN. May need continuation sheets or new prescription if space is filled up too quickly. The chart needs to be off the ward for compounding and release*
Intravenous fluid chart	Helps to establish a more accurate picture of total intravenous fluid prescribing, particularly for those staff reviewing for additional intravenous fluids with or without electrolytes	May not be sufficient room for detail of IVN. IVN prescriptions may become 'lost' following further intravenous fluid prescribing, particularly at weekends. Still need to look for fluid volumes and electrolytes from intravenous drugs on the medicine chart. The chart needs to be off the ward for compounding and release*
Dedicated IVN prescription chart	Allows sufficient detail to aid compounding and for ward staff about the IVN contents. The ownership of IVN prescribing more clearly lies with the nutrition team. Focus for information about patients prescribed IVN. Allows important additional preprinted information to be included on the prescription	Other staff may be less likely to look at this chart. May be lost on the ward – need to decide on a specific place to keep, such as with medicine chart or in a dedicated folder. Needs to be off the ward for compounding and release*

* Photocopying of prescriptions is undesirable due to changing prescriptions, confidentiality, storage and appropriate destruction of copies and so on.

Adult intravenous nutrition prescription

Patient name: _____		Consultant _____	Consultant team bleep _____	Ward _____
Hospital number: _____		Type of iv access for IVN _____	Central line tip position _____	Ward giving set type _____
Date of birth: _____		Prescribing notes:		

Nursing staff should confirm patient name, hospital number, bag batch number and date before administration. Any queries should be directed to the nutrition Support Team during normal working hours or to the emergency duty pharmacist outside normal working hours (via switchboard)

Date	Regimen	Bag contents (electrolytes in mmol)	Volume per 24 hours*	Rate and duration	Prescriber to sign	Stability	Technical services	Regimen release	Administer	Nurse to sign
	Name: Kcal: N (g): Volume (mL):	Na K Mg Ca	PO₄ Vitamins Trace elements	mL	mL/hour over hours			Batch Sign		Date Time	
	Name: Kcal: N (g): Volume (mL):	Na K Mg Ca	PO₄ Vitamins Trace elements	mL	mL/hour over hours			Batch Sign		Date Time	
	Name: Kcal: N (g): Volume (mL):	Na K Mg Ca	PO₄ Vitamins Trace elements	mL	mL/hour over hours			Batch Sign		Date Time	
	Name: Kcal: N (g): Volume (mL):	Na K Mg Ca	PO₄ Vitamins Trace elements	mL	mL/hour over hours			Batch Sign		Date Time	
	Name: Kcal: N (g): Volume (mL):	Na K Mg Ca	PO₄ Vitamins Trace elements	mL	mL/hour over hours			Batch Sign		Date Time	

* Note that only a proportion of the bag contents may be intended for administration

Figure 11.4 Example of a dedicated intravenous nutrition prescription chart.

- *Are further additions required to a regimen compounded in unlicensed Technical Services facilities (UK, see Chapter 15)?* If a regimen is compounded in an unlicensed Technical Services unit then no further additions should be made because of the microbiological risk of using a starting component that has not been terminally sterilised. The starting component would also be unlicensed.

Clinical compromise when prescribing IVN is not about compromise to patient care but about being skilled in the use of regimens that may not have been used otherwise. It is always important to make practical decisions where appropriate, whilst avoiding clinically unacceptable compromise.

Where to prescribe your regimen

When you come to write your IVN prescriptions there are several choices of documentation (Table 11.5), although a dedicated IVN prescription is most likely to be the appropriate option.

If using a dedicated IVN prescription chart, it is important to consider whether you will use computer-generated or hand-written prescriptions (Figure 11.3).

The format of dedicated prescription charts can vary widely depending on local needs, although the example shown in Figure 11.4 is a useful starting point.

Whichever type of IVN prescription you use, remember to keep the information updated as necessary. For example, if the patient transfers to another ward you will need to ensure that the correct regimen for the correct patient is delivered to the correct ward.

12

Complications of intravenous nutrition

Introduction

Intravenous nutrition (IVN) can cause a range of complications, including traumatic, infective, thrombotic and metabolic problems. At best, these require skill and resources to overcome whereas at worst they can be fatal. On some occasions, potential risks can also prevent IVN use when otherwise it would be indicated. Close clinical supervision and adequate monitoring are the only way to ensure early detection of problems in order to limit risks. All staff dealing with IVN patients must therefore understand IVN-related complications and teaching other staff to recognise the problems is an essential role for nutrition teams.

Complications of intravenous catheter insertion

Insertion of catheters for IVN (see Chapter 3) carries some immediate risk. This is dependent on the type of line involved, the skill of the professional placing it and the clinical condition of the patient. Most IVN catheters are placed using a Seldinger technique with a strict aseptic protocol to minimise infective risks (Figure 12.1).

It is often possible to place short-term IVN catheters on hospital wards but those for longer-term use, e.g. tunnelled lines, are usually placed in operating theatres. Patients with poor veins may also require line placement in theatre with Doppler vein imaging and/or cutdown techniques. Very difficult access is often best left to interventional radiologists.

The placement of central lines in subclavian or internal jugular veins carries more risk than peripheral catheter placement. Problems with arterial puncture, bleeding, pneumothorax and malposition can occur. Arterial puncture is usually obvious at the time of line insertion due to the high pressure and the presence of 'artery-red', pulsatile blood in the catheter. Nevertheless, there have been cases of IVN administration into arteries, which can cause limb discomfort if infused into a

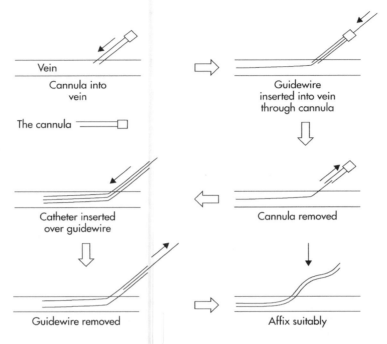

Vein

Cannula into vein

The cannula

Guidewire inserted into vein through cannula

Cannula removed

Catheter inserted over guidewire

Guidewire removed

Affix suitably

Figure 12.1 Intravenous line insertion using a Seldinger technique.

subclavian vessel and focal neurological symptoms or signs if infused into a carotid artery.

Placement of both subclavian and internal jugular catheters risks local bleeding. If the source of blood loss is the jugular vein, it is usually obvious and relatively easy to staunch with local pressure. However, bleeding from the subclavian may be unseen and not so easy to stop. The jugular approach is therefore favoured if the patient has any clotting abnormality.

Risks of accidental pneumothorax are also greater with subclavian insertions compared with internal jugular placements and, if an accidental pneumothorax would pose a very high risk for a patient, the subclavian route should be avoided (or only used with radiological or Doppler guidance). A chest X-ray is needed in all patients after upper-body central catheter placement to exclude a pneumothorax and to confirm the position of the catheter tip (see below). In order to avoid the serious dangers of bilateral pneumothoraces, a failed subclavian placement should be followed by X-ray exclusion of a pneumothorax *before* attempting the subclavian approach on the other side. Rarely, pneumothoraces are accompanied by significant surgical emphysema, with air under the skin causing swelling of the upper torso, neck or face. This crackles under the fingers when touched. Air embolus can also occur with central line or peripherally inserted central catheter (PICC) placement, since the high blood flow in central vessels can pull significant quantities of air into the circulation if the catheter is accidentally left open to the atmosphere.

Postplacement chest X-ray of a central catheter is also needed to confirm the position of the line tip. Routine placement of any central catheters without imaging cannot guarantee that the tip is in the correct position and problems such as cardiac arrhythmias arise if the line is in too far. Conversely, there is an increased risk of large-vein thrombosis if it is not in far enough. The catheter tip can also end up in the wrong vein, e.g. going up into the cerebral venous drainage rather than down towards the heart. Chest X-ray confirmation should be clearly documented by a clinician before the line is used. X-ray confirmation of correct tip position is not required for femoral lines.

If the line has been inserted too far, aseptic withdrawal is acceptable. However, if the catheter has not been inserted far enough, pushing it in further is not permissible since this may introduce infection from micro-organisms contaminating the catheter surface. Nevertheless, you can try to replace a line that is not in far enough by railroading a new one into the vein over a sterile guidewire placed through the original, badly positioned line before removal. A repeat chest-X ray is then required.

Complications from peripheral insertion of midline feeding catheters or peripheral feeding cannulae are usually local and minor. Placement should still use aseptic techniques and success is very dependent on the condition of the patient's veins. Midlines and peripheral cannulae do not need confirmation of correct placement prior to use, whereas PICC lines need to be treated the same as other central catheters.

Infective complications from intravenous nutrition

Catheter-related sepsis (CRS) is one of the commonest complications of IVN and reduction in CRS rates is a key goal for nutrition teams (see Chapter 14). CRS usually occurs from blood-borne bacterial infections following infection of an internal lumen of the feeding catheter from poor aseptic technique during catheter access. All catheter use should therefore be minimised and strict aseptic protocols must be used whenever the catheter is accessed for IVN, drug administration or blood sampling. Occasionally, a catheter is contaminated during insertion and skin infections at catheter exit sites can also track down to the blood stream.

CRS causes several symptoms and signs (Box 12.1) but it is often difficult to know whether a patient with apparent CRS problems actually has another source of infection. If the patient is obviously septic, investigations will be needed to determine the source. This requires various samples to be sent for culture, including urine, blood and, if appropriate, sputum or wound swabs. Imaging, for example, a chest X-ray or abdominal computerised tomography (CT), may also be required to exclude pneumonia or intra-abdominal collections. However, while results are pending, 'blind' treatment can be started to cover the most likely cause of infection.

Since IVN is an ideal growth medium for many micro-organisms, it is inappropriate to infuse feed through an infected line until the infection is at least controlled, if not eradicated, and all IVN should be discontinued whenever CRS is suspected. Resolution of pyrexia on cessation of feeding increases the likelihood that CRS was the problem. Carefully labelled (e.g. 'white lumen') blood cultures should be taken in all cases from each lumen, ideally with simultaneous peripheral blood cultures. Results take up to 48 hours to return and CRS is only unequivocally confirmed if a blood culture taken through one of the catheter lumens is not only positive but yields a colony count 1000 times greater than that from a simultaneous peripheral blood culture. If both peripheral and catheter cultures are not available, it is more difficult to be certain of CRS. A positive lumen culture with negative peripheral cultures suggests CRS is the problem but may be caused by sample

---

Box 12.1 Common signs of sepsis

General clinical deterioration
Rigors
Raised temperature $\geq 38°C$
Low temperature $\leq 36°C$
Raised pulse rate
Raised respiratory rate
Raised white cell count (occasionally low white count)
Raised inflammatory markers, e.g. C-reactive protein

contamination. A positive peripheral culture with either negative catheter cultures or catheter cultures with a similar colony count to that obtained peripherally suggests a non-catheter source of sepsis.

If CRS is not thought to be the likely cause of infection in an IVN patient, the line may still be used for feeding subject to regular review. If CRS is thought to be the problem in a short-term line, it should usually be removed and the tip sent for culture (the exit site must be disinfected before removal). Antibiotic treatment can then be given if necessary and the line replaced if needed once antibiotics are circulating. However, there is some risk of sepsis 'seeding' to a new catheter. Its use for IVN should therefore be avoided if possible until antibiotics have been given for 24–48 hours and appear to have been effective. Ideally, it is best to defer replacement of a catheter removed for suspected sepsis for this period if possible.

If CRS is suspected in a line needed for long-term access (e.g. a tunnelled line) or replacement of a short-term line would be very difficult or impractical, you can try to salvage the catheter from infection. When this is necessary, IVN should still be stopped and antibiotics commenced, usually beginning with 'blind' therapy (Box 12.2) and later modified following blood culture results.

If antibiotics are used to try to salvage an infected central line with more than one lumen, they should be given via alternate lumens for each dose. The last part of each dose should then be locked into the lumen until it is to be used again. This will discourage septic seeding between lumens. Some centres also use specific concentrated line locks for treatment of CRS, aiming for higher antimicrobial concentrations and so better clearance rates. We do not recommend this approach since the

---

Box 12.2 Typical 'blind' treatment of suspected intravenous nutrition line sepsis

Likely micro-organism:
Staphylococcus aureus (from skin)

Drugs of choice (in order of preference, depending on allergies and local policy):

1. Flucloxacillin (avoid, as there is a risk of methicillin-resistant *Staphylococcus aureus*)
2. Vancomycin
3. Teicoplanin
4. Linezolid

concentrations in the catheter achieved with conventional doses far exceed minimum inhibitory concentrations and it is important to ensure that the antibiotic is given in a volume that will permit adequate treatment of blood-borne infection.

Infected IVN catheters left in place for attempted salvage can, if absolutely necessary, be used for intravenous fluids and drugs, although this makes it difficult to lock antibiotics into the lumen(s). Furthermore, if absolutely necessary, a previously infected short-term line can also be used to recommence IVN if sepsis has been controlled for 24–48 hours by appropriate antibiotics which are going to be continued to complete a full treatment course. However, this practice will make complete clearance of a line infection less likely and hence should be avoided whenever attempting to salvage an infected long-term catheter (i.e. no IVN should be given during antimicrobial treatment for suspected or confirmed CRS in a long-term IVN line). It is also important that if any patient shows signs of worsening or renewed sepsis when recommencing IVN, it is immediately stopped and further cultures sent as above.

Other measures to help clear infection from long-term catheters include drugs to dissolve lipid or fibrinaceous deposits in which infection can persist (see below). Eradication of fungal line infections is particularly difficult and any use of the line during attempted treatment is always inadvisable. Sepsis related to a peripheral feeding line should always prompt immediate cessation of IVN and removal of the midline/cannula with the midline tips sent for culture.

Prophylaxis against internal lumen sepsis

The administration of antibiotics down a previously used line lumen to prepare it for IVN is unlikely to be effective and there is a risk of promoting bacterial resistance. Patients receiving long-term IVN as an intermittent infusion who have repeated CRS episodes may benefit from the use of prophylactic intravenous taurolidine. This is usually locked into the line lumen as a 2% solution after completing a feed and then flushed through before the next bag of IVN is commenced[1].

Occlusive catheter complications

Occlusion of a catheter prevents its use and the break-up of any solid material can risk embolisation, vein blockage and thrombosis. Occlusion results from a range of factors, shown in Box 12.3.

Box 12.3 Potential causes of intravenous catheter occlusion

Mechanical obstruction
- Closed clamp
- Kink in line
- Line tip against vein wall

Pharmacological incompatibility
- Intravenous nutrition instability
- Drug–drug precipitate
- Drug–nutrient precipitate

Deposition
- Lipid

Thrombosis
- In the central veins
- In the line lumen
- At the line tip

Whenever a catheter seems to be blocked, you should first check that there is no obvious mechanical obstruction such as a kinked line or closed tap. Establishing that the catheter tip is lying against the vein wall is difficult but is likely if repositioning of the patient allows free catheter flow. Imaging may be needed to confirm your suspicions.

If you think that the lumen itself is blocked, consider whether any therapies that could cause precipitation have been given. Any drug that is incompatible with cations such as magnesium or calcium, for example ciprofloxacin, will also be incompatible with IVN, and many other drugs can cause precipitation problems, e.g. aciclovir[2]. Sodium and/or fluid may destabilise the lipid in IVN and lipid deposition should be suspected if intravenous fluids, with or without electrolytes, have been run simultaneously with the IVN through the same lumen (see Appendix 1). Administration of blood or blood products with IVN should always be avoided for, although IVN is administered into the blood stream, there is inevitable uncertainty about its compatibility with non-blood components of blood products. Concentrations of electrolytes will also be much higher when the IVN and blood product mix within the catheter lumen compared to their mixing within a rapidly flowing vein. The same reasoning means that you should avoid putting incompatible therapies down the same lumen using devices such as a three-way tap or a side-infusion through a giving-set port, while you can allow them to be given down separate but adjacent lumens in

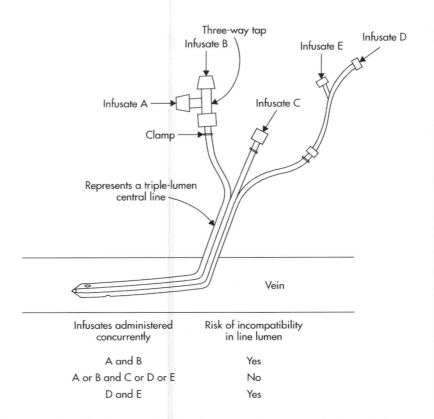

Figure 12.2 Risk of interaction of infusates used concurrently through the same intravenous line.

a central line, since rapid dilution will occur within the blood stream (Figure 12.2).

During prolonged IVN, lipid deposition can occur on the internal surface of catheters and this can also cause complete occlusion. Similarly, thrombosis can block catheters, especially if there has been any stagnation. Lines should therefore be flushed and locked between use and once-weekly alcohol locks to dissolve any lipid deposits should be considered in long-term IVN patients (see below).

Even when no stagnation occurs, fibrin clots can form on the line tip. These may cause a 'trapdoor' effect, allowing the line to be flushed through with ease but making it difficult to draw back blood (Figure 12.3).

Fibrin deposits on line tips can also extend to form large clots, which may occlude the vein and even embolise. It is therefore important

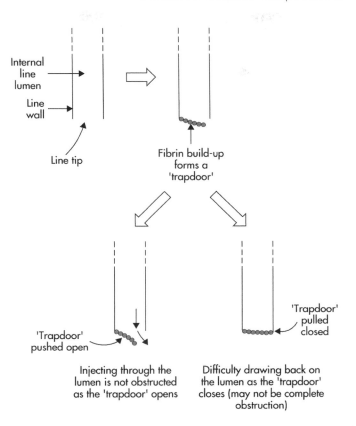

Internal
line
lumen

Line
wall

Line tip

Fibrin build-up
forms a
'trapdoor'

'Trapdoor'
pushed open

'Trapdoor'
pulled
closed

Injecting through the
lumen is not obstructed
as the 'trapdoor' opens

Difficulty drawing back on
the lumen as the 'trapdoor'
closes (may not be complete
obstruction)

Figure 12.3 Fibrin clot 'trapdoor' effect at the tip of an intravenous catheter.

to recognise signs of a developing problem such as difficulty drawing back on the line or partial obstruction. A large cuff of clot may also form around the line as it lies within a vein and if this is suspected, e.g. from arm swelling on the same side as a subclavian catheter, anticoagulation should be commenced immediately unless there is a major contraindication. Short-term lines should be removed, although in doing so there will be a small risk of precipitating a pulmonary embolus. With long-term lines, it may be appropriate to see whether the clot resolves with anticoagulation or even to use fibrinolytics. Venography may be needed to establish the extent and level of threat from a clotting problem and clearly, in some patients, the first recognition of a line-related clot will be a pulmonary embolus.

Prophylaxis against line occlusion

Prevention of catheter occlusion is clearly better than trying to clear an established blockage. Catheters should always be flushed before locking the line to limit any potential for coagulation. If, in order to prevent blood sample contamination, it is necessary to leave the IVN static in a lumen for a short period while the sample is taken from a different lumen, a flush should be given immediately after to all other lumens of the same line (never disconnect and reconnect an IVN bag). If an IVN bag runs out before the next one is available, it should be taken down promptly and the lumen flushed (see Chapter 16).

Several measures, related to the potential causes of line blockage (Box 12.3), can be helpful:

- Always manipulate and secure the line carefully
- Dedicate a lumen for IVN whenever possible
- Always be sure of compatibility before putting any other infusate through a catheter lumen at the same time as IVN (Figure 12.2; see Chapter 3 and Appendix 1)
- Always flush the lumen before a new IVN bag and between each IVN bag and each and every drug
- Do not leave IVN or blood products static in the lumen
- Use a push-pause technique to achieve greater turbulence within the lumen when flushing lines[3]
- Always report any stiffness in drawing back on a lumen – to detect tip thrombosis as early as possible
- Always report chest pain in the patient to a clinician since this may be due to vein thrombosis and embolisation

Catheter occlusion is a significant problem in patients on long-term home IVN, especially as many receive overnight infusions with the line left unused during the day[4]. A number of additional measures may be helpful in such patients:

- Heparin 'locking' of the IVN catheter during the day is advocated by some centres but is of uncertain effectiveness[4]
- Addition of heparin into IVN regimens[4] is used by some centres but may also be ineffective and may cause stability problems (Appendix 1, Box A1.4) whilst increasing bleeding risks
- Prophylactic alcohol locks are used by some centres to limit lipid deposition (Box 12.4)

Box 12.4 Prophylactic alcohol line locking

Indication
Limiting lumen lipid deposits where the patient receives long-term intravenous nutrition lipid

Method
Once-weekly instillation of 80% alcohol into the line lumen, left for 5 minutes before withdrawal. The volume instilled should be the volume of the lumen (ask manufacturer) plus a very small excess

Preparing 80% alcohol from 100% alcohol (also called absolute ethanol or dehydrated alcohol BP)

Take 4 mL of 100% alcohol and *make up to 5 mL* with water for injection. More than 1 mL of water for injection will be required

Cautions
Patient taking metronidazole or particularly disulfiram. Any other circumstances where alcohol is cautioned or contraindicated

---

- Reduction in the duration of lipid infusion in patients on long-term IVN[5]
- Twice-weekly administration of lipids (see Chapter 10)

Management of catheter occlusion

If a catheter does become occluded, the management depends on the most likely cause of the blockage (Box 12.5 and Table 12.1).

Thrombophlebitis

Thrombophlebitis refers to inflammation of a vein wall. It can be painful, will predispose to thrombosis and can make a vein unusable in the future. Central vein thrombophlebitis is uncommon due to the dilutional effect of the fast blood flow but it may occur when the tip of the catheter rests directly on the vein wall. This causes both trauma and a high local concentration of infusate. It is usually manifest by central aching pain, made worse when IVN is being infused.

Peripheral vein thrombophlebitis (PVT) is relatively common with midlines and very common with peripheral cannulae. The use of peripheral cannulae for the administration of IVN is therefore discouraged

---

Box 12.5 Management options for central line occlusion, numbered in usual order of preference for suspected cases

Mechanical obstruction
1 Check line for kinks

Pharmaceutical instability

Soluble in acidic conditions (e.g. etoposide or heparin with amikacin or vancomycin[6]):
1 Acid

Soluble in alkaline conditions (e.g. phenytoin[3])
1 Sodium bicarbonate

Lipid deposition
1 Alcohol
2 Acid
3 Fibrinolytic

Thrombosis
1 Fibrinolytic
2 Alcohol
3 Acid

Further details of management options can be found in Table 12.1

---

unless staff resources allow the cannula used to be swapped to a different vein after every IVN bag (see below). Signs of peripheral thrombophlebitis are shown in Box 12.6. Severe local damage related to thrombophlebitis can lead to tissue necrosis (Plate 4).

Box 12.6 Signs of peripheral vein thrombophlebitis

Local (i.e. same limb)
Erythema (redness)
Swelling
Inflammation
Pain
Soreness
Aching

Remember that the tip of a midline may be some distance from the apparent vein entry site

---

Table 12.1 Details of management options for central line occlusion*

Management option	Details	Examples of variations and notes
Acid	0.1 molar hydrochloric acid instilled into the lumen, left for up to 1 hour**, then withdrawn and repeated if necessary	0.1% hydrochloric acid[3], 0.1 N hydrochloric acid[6,7]
Alcohol	80% alcohol instilled into the lumen, left for up to 1 hour**, then withdrawn and repeated if necessary	Other concentrations of alcohol may be recommended – 70%[3,7] or 90%[4]
Fibrinolytic	Urokinase 5000 units per mL[6,3,8] or Streptokinase 250 units per mL[8] instilled into the lumen, left for 1 hour**, then withdrawn and repeated if necessary	Avoid use of streptokinase; consider alteplase first. Adverse effects are more likely with streptokinase than with urokinase[3,8] and there is a risk of sensitisation and ineffectiveness if previously treated with streptokinase. The recommended urokinase dwell time may vary – 5–10 minutes[8], 30–60 minutes[3], 2 hours[6]. The use of an infusion[4,9] is not recommended due to the risks of forcing solid material into the vein and rupturing the line. Forcing the catheter lumen may cause rupture[10] and this may force solid material into the vein
Sodium bicarbonate	1 mEq/ml sodium bicarbonate instilled into the lumen, left for up to 1 hour**, then withdrawn and repeated if necessary	Do not use with intravenous nutrition precipitation because calcium and phosphate solubility is pH-dependent[6], being higher at low pH and adding more bicarbonate increases the pH, which is likely to lead to further precipitation/solidification[6]

 * Note that for all lumen instillations the volume instilled should be the volume of the lumen (ask manufacturer) plus a very small excess.

** Check compatibility with line manufacturer and refer to local guide lines.

Table 12.2 Risk factors for intravenous nutrition (IVN)-related thrombophlebitis

Risk factor	Reasons
Small vein diameter	Small veins have low blood flow and hence there is relatively less dilution of the hypertonic IVN[11,12]
External diameter of intravenous catheter	Small intravenous catheters permit higher rates of blood flow around them and hence greater dilution of administered IVN[11]. They are also less likely to cause direct irritation of vein walls
IVN concentration	Higher IVN concentrations are more likely to cause tonicity-related damage to cells lining the veins
Inherent venous irritability of IVN components	Potassium is an example of a component that is inherently irritant to veins
Condition of veins	Frail and elderly patients often have less patent veins with lower tolerance to vein trauma. Veins recently used for previous venepuncture or fluid administration may have some existing damage, predisposing to thrombophlebitis
Duration of IVN administration	The longer a vein is used, the more likely that irritation and damage will occur

A variety of risk factors predispose to the development of PVT (Table 12.2).

Prophylaxis against peripheral vein thrombophlebitis

Several measures may help to reduce the incidence or severity of PVT (Box 12.7), although the success of pharmacological prophylaxis against PVT is probably limited[16]. The use of multiple techniques may offer benefit when giving IVN via a midline[17] although, in our and other's experience, midline IVN is often well tolerated anyway, even if using IVN osmolalities usually intended for central rather than peripheral administration[18].

Some groups have also reported success using peripheral cannulae for IVN with no pharmacological interventions other than low regimen osmolality, as long as the IVN is administered as an intermittent infusion for 12 hours in 24, removing and replacing the cannula in the opposite arm (avoiding the anticubital veins) for each bag[14]. However, the use of this technique requires impeccable cannula care and considerable

---

Box 12.7 Potential measures to help prevent peripheral vein thrombophlebitis

Addition of hydrocortisone and/or heparin to the intravenous nutrition (IVN) regimen

Topical 5 mg glyceryl trinitrate patch

Topical non-steroidal anti-inflammatory drug to appropriate limb[13]

Limiting duration of IVN administration through a peripheral cannula before replacement[14,15]

Using a midline rather than a peripheral cannula

Limiting concentration of IVN regimens (do not use lipid-free regimens peripherally due to the high osmolality of the glucose). This may require a significant compromise on nitrogen and energy provision

Always ensure adequate stability data before adding anything to an IVN regimen (e.g. the addition of hydrocortisone and heparin to regimens may cause problems[11])

---

resources to ensure prompt resiting of the cannulas. Repeated cannula replacement is also painful for patients[15].

Plate 4 shows unexpected tissue necrosis as a result of a peripheral micronutrient infusion through a cannula – a warning of the consequences of using too high a concentration in too small a vein.

Management of peripheral vein thrombophlebitis

When PVT is suspected, IVN should be discontinued and the catheter removed. The tip of the line (excluding peripheral cannulae) should then be sent for culture. Persistent pain caused by PVT may be helped by the topical application of a corticosteroid (e.g. 1% w/w hydrocortisone) to the affected site.

Microparticulate risks of intravenous nutrition and in-line filtration

An in-line filter (attached to the IVN giving set) acts as a sieve, preventing any contaminants larger than the filter pore size entering the patient's vein (Box 12.8). The use of such filters is recommended by some authorities with a view to reducing a number of potential problems, including the incidence of PVT. However, the use of filters, although

---

Box 12.8 Examples of potential intravenous nutrition contaminants removed by in-line filtration

Particulates shed from the internal surfaces of the bag and giving set

Glass particles introduced from bag additions from glass ampoules

Precipitates in case of compounding errors or inappropriate bag storage

Large lipid globules from 'creaming' (see Appendix 1) or bulk lipid infusions

Microbiological contaminants such as fungi or endotoxins

Note
Contaminant retention depends on the specific filter characteristics, e.g. the pore size used. For regimens with lipid this is 1.2 micron to allow the lipid globules through. For lipid-free regimens it is 0.2 micron. Other filter characteristics can include charged coatings which aid retention of endotoxins and allow longer use of the filter (refer to manufacturer's recommendations and local policy)

---

desirable, comes at a significant cost and, although the intravenous infusion of any large pieces of solid material is a definite risk for problems such as pulmonary embolus, it is more difficult to provide evidence that limiting infusion of the tiny particulates shown in Box 12.8 grants significant advantages. Furthermore, most short-term IVN patients are likely to receive many other infusions without in-line filtration, all of which pose the same potential problem of microparticulate infusion. Retention of fungi, the other proposed argument for in-line filters, is also unlikely to be an issue given that IVN compounding facilities (see Chapter 15) are designed to prevent microbiological contamination of prepared bags. These facilities should also routinely filter injections drawn from glass ampoules to limit glass particles. We therefore recommend that the use of in-line filtration is reserved for patients on long-term IVN (plus infants and small children), although such advice does add a risk management aspect to the IVN service.

If an appropriately sized filter is being used and it blocks, it should never be removed to continue the infusion. This is because the blockage must be assumed to be due to clogging with contaminants that have been prevented from entering the patient's veins. Stop and disconnect the IVN infusion and seek specialist advice from the nutrition team or Technical Services (see Chapter 15).

Metabolic complications of intravenous nutrition

Metabolic complications of IVN usually result from inadequate, excessive or unbalanced provision of individual IVN components (see Chapters 7–10). The most common metabolic problem is hyperglycaemia, whereas the most dangerous is the refeeding syndrome (see Chapters 8 and 9). Allergic reactions to the lipid component of IVN have also been reported but are rare[19].

Complications related to fluid

Fluid overload, especially with saline, can result in oedema, congestive cardiac failure and worsening ascites. It can also precipitate partial ileus or delay the recovery of gut function following abdominal surgery. It may therefore contribute to the original need for IVN and then prolong that need. Overload with hypotonic fluids can also cause dilution of plasma with widespread effects, including cardiorespiratory compromise, hyponatraemia, confusion and even coma. Fluid deficiency results in dehydration with multiple potential consequences. These include reduced blood pressure and cardiac output, concentration of serum electrolytes with pseudohypernatraemia, nausea, vomiting, confusion, coma and renal failure. More details of these fluid-related problems are given in Chapters 7 and 10.

Excessive or inadequate provision of amino acids

Excess provision of amino acids is not usually considered harmful and, within limits, may improve nitrogen balance. As discussed in Chapter 7, however, the pattern of amino acids provided by IVN may not be fully utilised by sick patients who need an unusual pattern to meet the demands of their acute-phase response. High levels of amino acid provision may therefore produce metabolic upset (see Chapter 7) and will also result in increased urea production that will need to be cleared by the kidneys (see Chapter 10).

Inadequate provision of amino acids will result in excessive lean tissue loss.

Excessive or inadequate provision of carbohydrate

High levels of glucose provision cause hyperglycaemia, not only in previously diabetic patients, but also in many seriously ill or injured patients who are frequently insulin-resistant. This can have several serious consequences, including:

- Increased risk of sepsis
- Increased risk of rebound hypoglycaemia on stopping IVN
- Higher probability of refeeding syndrome
- Diabetic ketoacidosis
- Increased carbon dioxide production (see Chapter 10)
- When administering IVN through peripheral veins, an increased risk of thrombophlebitis
- Abnormal liver function

Inadequate provision of glucose in IVN may result in hypoglycaemia and a low total calorific intake will cause weight loss as well as limiting the capacity to utilise amino acids in the IVN for protein manufacture. Prescribing IVN for diabetics or those patients with insulin resistance is considered in Chapter 10.

Excessive or inadequate provision of lipid

Excessive provision of lipids in IVN can result in respiratory compromise and coagulopathies[20]. In the long term, it may also cause liver damage (see below) and could be a risk for atheroma. The respiratory compromise from excess lipid includes both an increased infective risk due to lipid accumulation in macrophages, especially in the lung, and the problems of increased oxygen demands due to the greater need for oxygen when metabolising lipid compared to glucose for the same amount of energy production (see Chapter 10).

Inadequate lipid provision in IVN can result in low total energy provision and hence weight loss. In the longer term it may also lead to deficiency of essential fatty acids, including ω_6-linoleic acid and ω_3-linolenic acids needed for membrane function and immune/inflammatory responses (see Chapter 7). Inadequate lipid energy also increases the osmolality of the IVN due to the additional glucose and hence the risk of thrombophlebitis if administered into a peripheral vein (see above and Chapter 7).

Excessive or inadequate provision of electrolytes

Abnormalities in plasma or tissue electrolyte levels may cause severe problems (see Chapter 8) and disturbances of sodium, potassium, calcium, magnesium and phosphate are frequently seen in IVN patients.

They are particularly common during the early stage of IVN when changes in whole-body electrolyte content due to the effects of malnourishment are coupled with the problems of abnormal electrolyte regulation, provision and loss that are so common in intestinal failure patients. They are also integral to the threat from refeeding syndrome which puts patients at grave risk (see Chapter 8).

Excessive or inadequate provision of micronutrients

Excessive or inadequate provision of micronutrients can result in the toxicity or deficiency problems described in Chapter 9. The development of Wernicke–Korsakoff syndrome with refeeding is a particular danger. There may also be interactions with other therapies, for example excessive vitamin K administration can result in difficulties obtaining a therapeutic international normalised ratio (INR) for patients requiring warfarin.

Liver function abnormalities

IVN can lead to both acute and long-term abnormalities in liver function. In the acute setting, it may be difficult to determine whether a liver problem is IVN-induced or whether it is due to other aspects of the patient's illness, including:

- Portal bacterial translocation (e.g. in hepatobiliary or pancreatic surgery patients and patients with intra-abdominal infection or small-bowel overgrowth)
- Sepsis from any source
- Biliary obstruction of any cause, e.g. retained stone
- Unrecognised previous chronic liver disease (e.g. long-term alcohol-related liver damage)
- New liver disease (e.g. drug reaction, infective hepatitis or liver abscess)

IVN patients with liver function abnormalities may therefore need imaging of the liver (usually starting with an ultrasound), blood tests for other causes of liver disease and a careful review of drug charts to check for possible side-effects from other drug therapy.

Most early (< 3 weeks) changes in liver function that are due to IVN are usually a consequence of steatosis (fatty liver). This usually causes a modest rise in level of alanine or aspartate transaminase (see Chapter 13). The abnormalities tend to occur in the first few days or weeks of IVN, especially if there is excess glucose provision and the patient has previously been very malnourished. There is usually little or no disturbance in liver synthetic function and the changes are generally of little concern[21].

The liver complications of longer-term IVN tend to be predominantly cholestatic (see Chapters 10 and 13). These usually occur several weeks or months into intravenous feeding and initially cause increases in alkaline phosphatase levels. Later there may be rising bilirubin and transaminase levels with significant impairment of liver synthetic function. The latter is best monitored by measuring INR. If unchecked, long-term IVN liver damage can occur with progress to cirrhosis and liver failure. It is particularly seen in home IVN patients who have been fed for several years (see Chapter 13).

Intrahepatic cholestasis is the commonest problem underlying the IVN-induced cholestatic changes and particularly occurs with overprovision of lipid. It can occur, however, with quite modest feeding levels in vulnerable individuals. The cause is unclear but may relate to the loss of neurohumoral signalling from the gastrointestinal tract to the liver, such as the absence of the normal cholecystokinin release triggered by meals. Cholestatic problems are particularly common in patients with a very short bowel and high stomal losses, possibly due to the high loss of bile salts from the stoma which leads to reduced bile solubility. Actual biliary sludging, acalculous cholecystitis, gallbladder dilatation and gallstones can occur in any long-term IVN patient, especially with excessive energy intake from glucose or lipid. These may result in significant biliary obstruction and hence further increase the risks of cirrhosis. Abnormal levels of bacterial translocation from a damaged gut via the portal system may also play a role in causing liver damage in some patients and it is worth trying a course of antibiotics (e.g. ciprofloxacin with metronidazole) likely to be active against a broad range of gastrointestinal organisms.

Management of IVN-induced liver dysfunction

If, after other potential causes have been excluded, the most likely cause of liver dysfunction appears to be the IVN, you will need to review and amend the prescription. A number of potential changes can be made but you will need to allow 10–14 days after each to determine whether they have led to any benefit. The following should be tried first:

- Review the patient's energy requirements (see Chapters 7 and 11) and, if lower than the total currently provided from *all routes*, reduce the IVN energy provision.
- Check that the ratio of glucose to lipid energy is as close to 50:50 as possible (see Chapter 7).
- Try intermittent IVN: gradually run the IVN regimen over a shorter duration using a higher rate, ultimately aiming to give over 12–16 hours with a significant physiological rest period (see Chapter 7).

If none of these measures helps, consider the following further options:

- Increase the relative glucose content – to give a glucose-to-lipid energy ratio of approximately 70:30. This type of regimen, with a high glucose content, will initially need to be given over 24 hours through a central vein with careful blood glucose monitoring.
- Switch to giving lipid in the IVN regimen on only 2 days per week, using glucose as the sole energy source on the remaining days.
- Change the type of lipid provided: different lipids may have less effect on the liver, although further evidence of this possibility is required (see Chapter 7).

In addition to the above measures, is also possible to consider oral ursodeoxycholic acid[22], although further studies are required to prove its efficacy for this indication.

Conclusions

IVN complications are many, varied and can frequently occur with potentially fatal results. Prescribing from an office without a nutritional review of the patient is therefore always inappropriate and it is critical to ensure close clinical and laboratory monitoring of all IVN patients.

References

1. Jurewitsch B, Lee T, Park J, Jeejeebhoy K. Taurolidine 2% as an antimicrobial lock solution for prevention of recurrent catheter-related bloodstream infections. *J Parenteral Enteral Nutr* 1998; 22: 242–244.
2. Trissel L. *Handbook on Injectable Drugs*. Bethseda: American Society of Health-System Pharmacists, 2005: 11.
3. Harris J, Maguire D. Developing a protocol to prevent and treat paediatric central venous catheter occlusions. *J Intravenous Nurs* 1999; 22: 194–198.
4. Williams N, Wales S, Scott N, Irving M. The incidence and management of catheter occlusion in patients on home parenteral nutrition. *Clin Nutr* 1993; 12: 344–349.

5. Beau P, Matuchansky C. Lipid delivery and catheter obstruction during cyclic total parenteral nutrition. *Lancet* 1987; 7: 1095–1096.

6. Shulman R, Reed T, Pitre D, Laine L. Use of hydrochloric acid to clear obstructed central venous catheters. *J Parenteral Enteral Nutr* 1988; 12: 509–510.

7. Werlin S, Lausten T, Jessen S et al. Treatment of central venous catheter occlusions with ethanol and hydrochloric acid. *J Parenteral Enteral Nutr* 1995; 19: 416–418.

8. Hurtubise M, Bottino J, Lawson M, McCredie K. Restoring patency of occluded central venous catheters. *Arch Surg* 1980; 115: 212–213.

9. Haire W, Lieberman R. Thrombosed central venous catheters: restoring function with 6-hour urokinase infusion after failure of bolus urokinase. *J Parenteral Enteral Nutr* 1992; 16: 129–132.

10. Mughal M. Complications of intravenous feeding catheters. *Br J Surg* 1989; 76: 15–21.

11. Payne-James J, Khawaja H. First choice for total parenteral nutrition: the peripheral route. *J Parenteral Enteral Nutr* 1993; 17: 468–478.

12. Everitt N, McMahon M. Influence of fine-bore catheter length on infusion thrombophlebitis in peripheral intravenous nutrition: a randomised controlled trial. *Ann R Coll Surg Engl* 1997; 79: 221–224.

13. Payne-James J, Bray M, Kapadia S et al. Topical nonsteroidal anti-inflammatory gel for the prevention of peripheral vein thrombophlebitis. *Anaesthesia* 1992; 47: 324–326.

14. May J, Murchan P, MacFie J et al. Prospective study of the aetiology of infusion phlebitis and line failure during peripheral parenteral nutrition. *Br J Surg* 1996; 83: 1091–1094.

15. Madan M, Alexander D, McMahon M. Influence of catheter type on occurrence of thrombophlebitis during peripheral intravenous nutrition. *Lancet* 1992; 339: 101–103.

16. Dobbins B, Catton J, Tighe M et al. Randomised clinical trials to determine the role of topical glyceryl trinitrate in peripheral intravenous nutrition. *Br J Surg* 2003; 90: 804–810.

17. Tighe M, Wong C, Martin I, McMahon M. Do heparin, hydrocortisone, and glyceryl trinitrate influence thrombophlebitis during full intravenous nutrition via a peripheral vein? *J Parenteral Enteral Nutr* 1995; 19: 507–509.

18. Kane K, Cologiovanni L, McKiernan J et al. High osmolality feedings do not increase the incidence of thrombophlebitis during peripheral iv nutrition. *J Parenteral Enteral Nutr* 1996; 20: 194–197.

19. Levy M, Dupuis L. Parenteral nutrition hypersensitivity. *J Parenteral Enteral Nutr* 1990; 14: 213–215.

20. Klein C, Stanek G, Wiles C. Overfeeding macronutrients to critically ill adults: metabolic complications. *J Am Dietetic Assoc* 1998; 98: 795–806.

21. Payne-James, Grimble G, Silk D, eds. *Artificial Nutrition Support in Clinical Practice*, 2nd edn. London: Greenwich Medical Media, 2001: 491–492.

22. Beau P, Labat-Labourdette J, Ingrand P, Beauchant M. Is ursodeoxycholic acid an effective therapy for total parenteral nutrition-related liver disease? *J Hepatol* 1994; 20: 240–244.

13

Monitoring

Introduction

In view of the potential risks outlined in Chapter 12, regular review and monitoring of intravenous nutrition (IVN) patients are essential. The aim is both to prevent complications and to recognise others as early as possible in order to limit their consequences. Regular review also allows you to amend the nutritional care plan to permit appropriate progress towards feeding by oral or enteral tube routes and so prevent overuse of IVN.

Both clinical and laboratory review are needed on a daily basis during the early stages of intravenous feeding but later, in longer-term, more stable IVN patients, monitoring can be far less frequent even though additional concerns arise (see below). Following your review, it is essential to document all decisions and consider whether other staff need to be informed of any important problems or regimen changes, e.g. the ward nursing staff, ward pharmacist, the patient's medical team or the dietitian. Summary tables modified from the National Institute for Health and Clinical Excellence (NICE) recommendations for laboratory monitoring for short-term IVN patients are given in Table 13.1.

Clinical monitoring of intravenous nutrition patients

In many ways, the clinical monitoring of patients on IVN is a brief repeat of their initial assessment (see Chapter 4). Any new history and a brief clinical examination are therefore needed along with a check of temperature, pulse, respiration, body weight, fluid balance, drug and food intake charts. However, since the patient has started IVN, all of these assessments now have the additional purpose of checking whether there is anything to suggest infective, thrombotic or metabolic complications. You therefore assess:

- Current general status and signs of infection
- Current gastrointestinal function

Table 13.1 Minimum requirements for short-term laboratory monitoring of patients requiring nutritional support*

Reported	Frequency		Notes
	To begin	Once stable†	
Sodium, potassium, urea, creatinine	Baseline then daily	1–3 times a week	See Chapters 8 and 10
Magnesium and phosphate	Baseline then daily	1–3 times a week	See Chapters 8 and 10
Calcium and albumin	Baseline then daily	1–3 times a week	See Chapters 8 and 10. Always correct plasma calcium for albumin
Glucose	Baseline then at least daily	1–3 times a week	See Chapter 10. Not usually required if having regular 'finger sticks' testing
Liver function, including international normalised ratio (INR)	Baseline then twice weekly	Weekly	See Chapters 10 and 12
C-reactive protein	Baseline then 2–3 times a week	Weekly	See Chapter 4
Full blood count	Baseline then 1–2 times a week	Weekly	See Chapter 4
Trace elements (zinc, selenium, copper, manganese)	Baseline if indicated	Every 2–4 weeks	See Chapter 9. Need to use a special metal-free sampling tube
Vitamins (A, D, E, B_{12} and folic acid)	Baseline if indicated, e.g. always check vitamin B_{12} and folic acid levels if terminal ileum missing	Every 2–4 weeks	See Chapter 9

* More extensive monitoring is required in unstable patients or those patients with other conditions requiring it. Interpret all reported results with care; see relevant chapters.

† If becomes unstable, return to 'to begin' monitoring. Long-term monitoring can be found in Chapter 13.

Modified from the National Institute for Health and Clinical Excellence (NICE) guidelines[1].

- Nutrient intake since the last review and current nutritional status
- Fluid balance since the last review and current fluid status
- IVN line or vein-related problems
- Metabolic abnormalities
- Current drug therapies

Once these are determined you can decide whether IVN should be continued, whether it is safe and practical to do so and whether the current regimen needs any alterations.

General status and signs of infection

A grasp of how well the patient is doing overall is a very important part of clinical care. It is obtained in part by looking at the notes and asking the ward and medical staff. However, above all it is obtained by looking and talking to the patient. An 'end-of-bed' perspective can often tell you as much or more than a careful examination and, in particular, one of the main purposes of seeing the patient is to ask yourself whether he or she is getting better or worse and whether, if the latter is the case, the deterioration could in any way be due to the IVN.

Examination of the temperature, pulse, blood pressure and respiration chart is also a critical part of a general assessment. In particular, it helps you decide whether there is any likelihood of sepsis, a suspicion that might be supported by increases in white blood cell count (WBC) and C-reactive protein (CRP). Confirmation and more specific diagnosis from results of blood or urine cultures etc. can then be made later. If sepsis seems likely, the actions described in Chapter 12 should be taken, bearing in mind the possibility of more than one focus of infection.

Gastrointestinal function

Deciding on whether the patient still has intestinal failure or continued inaccessibility of the gastrointestinal tract determines whether there is a continued need for IVN. Once again, the information you require can largely be derived from a check of the notes, quizzing the ward staff and asking the patient questions. Discussions with the patient's main care team are often useful and you may need to examine the patient's abdomen and review fluid charts (see below).

Your aim is to establish:

- Whether any oral or enteral intake is being permitted and if not, why the restriction remains
- Whether any oral or enteral intake is being tolerated without pain or nausea
- Whether the patient has been vomiting or has had high nasogastric tube aspirates
- Whether the patient has abdominal distension
- The volume and nature of any losses through abdominal drains or fistulae
- The volume and nature of faecal loss or the passage of wind via stomas or per rectum

Nutritional intake and nutritional status

Since the purpose of IVN is to ensure that the total nutrient intake meets the patient's requirements, you need to review any intake via oral and enteral routes as well as checking whether the IVN prescribed has actually been given as intended.

Many IVN patients are 'nil by mouth' or tube, but it is important to maintain intake charts for those who are eating or drinking, starting to do so, or receiving any enteral tube feeding. These charts should show everything nutritious that the patient receives but they are often unreliable. This is true for charts completed by patients themselves or by the ward staff. You therefore need to ask the patient, if possible, to confirm entries and to try to recall omissions. Be aware that records of a patient being offered food do not necessarily mean it was consumed. The same applies to oral sip supplements recorded on drug charts and, to a lesser extent, to tube feeds recorded on enteral feeding charts.

A review of the patient's IVN provision includes a check that the bag being administered is going at the correct rate for the correct duration, and that there have been no significant breaks in administration due to complications or logistic delays (e.g. no bag reaching the ward). It is particularly important to ensure that any delays in administration have not led to a compounded IVN bag being kept out at room temperature for longer than the manufacturer recommends (usually an absolute maximum of 48 hours).

Review of nutritional status does not require daily weighing and although a once- or twice-weekly weight chart does help to monitor nutritional balance and achievement of targets, it is only of value over longer periods since any acute weight changes are likely to be fluid-related (see below). A weekly clinical check for improvements in any symptoms or signs of specific nutrient deficiency (such as a sore mouth or skin rash) may clearly be of relevance.

Fluid balance and current fluid status

Frequent clinical assessments of fluid status, along with reviews of fluid balance charts and laboratory measurements of renal function (see below), are also a part of daily reassessment/monitoring during early IVN provision. This requires a brief examination for signs of dehydration or fluid overload, such as diminished skin turgor or oedema (see Chapter 4). A falling blood pressure with an increasing pulse rate can also be due to dehydration, although the combination can be a reflection of infection or bleeding. Rapid changes in body weight are invariably caused by changes in total body water and clinical assessments of jugular venous pressure, measurements of central venous pressure and a check for signs of pulmonary congestion (fine, bilateral chest crackles) are also helpful. Oedematous patients are very likely to have excess total body sodium as well as excess body water and so a reduction of sodium provision as well as fluid volume will often be desirable.

Plates 2a and 2b show the resolution of noticeable peripheral oedema over 6 days in a postsurgical patient. Scrotal oedema leads to significant discomfort and can be very painful. More importantly, oedema is usually associated with pulmonary congestion, which causes breathlessness and predisposes to pneumonia. Furthermore, peripheral oedema is associated with oedema of the gut, which can delay the re-establishment of oral or enteral nutrition.

As with food charts, fluid balance charts should record *all* inputs and outputs but are also frequently incomplete or inaccurate. You therefore need to check that fluid administration from all oral and enteral sources, i.e. food, drinks, sip feeds and tube feeds, and all intravenous sources, i.e. the IVN, other intravenous fluids and intravenous drugs (see Chapter 5), have been accounted for. All types of fluid loss must also be documented with careful attention to losses via naso-gastric tubes, drains and any significant diarrhoea or liquid stomal loss. You also need to recognise that, whereas all intravenous fluids produce a net gain in body water, fluids administered orally or enterally may not do so. A patient with a short bowel to a stoma, for example, may become dehydrated and sodium-depleted from drinking large quantities of oral fluid since the hypotonicity can draw salt and water into the upper small-bowel lumen and lead to excessive stomal loss (see Chapter 10).

The provision of electrolytes in the IVN or by other routes may be critically dependent on the volume and type of current fluid losses. For example, fluid losses from high small-bowel stomas or fistulae will be high in sodium (probably around 100 mmol/L) whereas large fluid losses due to nasogastric tube aspirates, vomiting or diarrhoea will be high in potassium. You must therefore account for these potential losses in your prescribing.

Intravenous nutrition line problems

Your clinical review of IVN patients should also include a review of any line-related problems (see Chapter 12).

The giving sets and the catheter itself should be inspected for any kinks or damage (Plates 7a and 7b) and you should see that the line is securely fixed to the skin and covered with an appropriate dressing. There are many suitable dressings available but ideally a transparent, semipermeable covering should be used which allows a view of the line site to check for problems such as infection, while preventing build-up of moisture which can encourage microbiological growth. Dressings should be replaced promptly if they become loose or soiled.

The catheter exit site should be checked for any local infection and should be swabbed for culture if present. Any likely problems with thrombophlebitis or thrombosis must be identified with checks for any redness, swelling or pain. This can be related to either the immediate course of the vein in which a peripheral catheter is placed or, for both peripheral and central catheters, the region of vein drainage.

Maintaining a viable central line is particularly important when it is a tunnelled line because of the long-term implications of repeated line failure. Additionally these lines tend to hang down further, making them more vulnerable to contamination from stomas or open wounds. They should always be kept away from such dangers and may require either careful looping under the dressing or to be loosely tied up to reduce the exposure of the line to infection hazards.

Drug therapies

Changes in any drugs the patient may be taking can affect your IVN prescription. For example, the introduction of amphotericin is likely to cause increased renal potassium loss[2] and hence the need for additional supplementation. Starting some intravenous antibiotics will contribute large amounts of sodium and hence decrease IVN requirements. Checking for non-administration of medicines is also important. The reason for drugs not being given may prompt a change in the drug or its formulation and very occasionally moving to administer it within the IVN can be appropriate if stability issues allow it. If any drugs are used to try to improve tolerance to peripherally administered IVN, e.g. a glyceryl trinitrate patch, the specialised nature of the indication must be clearly documented on the medicine chart so that the therapy is not continued indefinitely.

Laboratory monitoring in the acute setting

The need for haematological, biochemical and microbiological monitoring of your patients depends on their clinical and nutritional status. Patients who have just commenced IVN should always be considered relatively unstable due to the potential for refeeding syndromes and the large variation in tolerance to intravenously administered macronutrients, fluids and electrolytes.

All access of IVN catheters, including access for blood sampling, must be carried out using the strictest aseptic technique to minimise infective risk. This includes other lumens of the same central line because of the potential for cross-contamination or 'seeding' into the IVN lumen. Whenever possible, it should therefore remain normal practice to take peripheral blood for haematology and biochemistry monitoring rather than taking the samples from a central line. However, this may not be practical in a patient with poor peripheral veins.

When taking central line blood samples for laboratory analysis, any IVN running through another lumen must be briefly stopped to avoid drawing up concentrated lipid or electrolytes into the sample tube. Although it is the first blood from the line that is required for microbiological culture, the first 10 mL should be discarded for haematology or biochemistry analysis. Specialist tubes may be required for particular tests (e.g. metal-free tubes for trace element levels).

Ensuring minimum standards for laboratory monitoring of patients is important to ensure that you are prescribing what the patient requires and that any complications (see Chapter 12) are detected at the earliest opportunity. Table 13.1 shows minimum recommended monitoring for patients who require nutritional review or support regardless of the method of feeding, i.e. oral, enteral tube or intravenous.

Monitoring haematology

A daily full blood count is usually appropriate during the early days of IVN. A fall in haemoglobin usually indicates blood loss or haemolysis, although if it occurs slowly in longer-term patients, inadequate iron provision or, more rarely, other problems such as inadequate copper must be considered. A rapid increase in haemoglobin without preceding transfusion may be due to haemoconcentration secondary to inadequate fluids.

A rising WBC is of particular importance as a marker of potential infection and the possibility of catheter-related sepsis (CRS). It can, however, be difficult to interpret in IVN patients who often have multiple potential reasons for a rise. A low WBC is a frequent finding in chemotherapy patients, especially haemato-oncology patients who have received high-dose chemotherapy for bone marrow malignancies and who need the IVN because of collateral gut damage (see Chapter 3). Occasionally, a low WBC is seen in longer-term IVN patients who develop antibodies which damage white cells, probably from immune responses to the lipid component of their IVN.

Monitoring blood glucose

Monitoring of blood glucose is initially needed four times daily in IVN patients, with even more frequent measures in patients known to be diabetic and those who develop raised glucose levels with feeding. Ward measures such as BM Stix are used with records kept on specific blood glucose monitoring charts. Levels consistently above 11 mmol/L should prompt the introduction of insulin initially on a sliding scale and tighter control is exercised on many intensive care units (see Chapter 10). Insulin-dependent diabetic patients should always be commenced on a sliding scale when IVN is started. Low rebound blood glucose values may occur when IVN is stopped and, for this reason, it is common practice to reduce rates to 50% for a short period before stopping IVN altogether.

Monitoring inflammatory markers

Rises in the levels of CRP and, to a lesser, extent erythrocyte sedimentation rate are often used as early indicators of CRS although, as with rising WBCs, most IVN patients have many potential reasons for a rise.

Monitoring electrolytes and renal function

The acute monitoring of electrolytes and renal function includes not only daily measurement of the routine sodium, potassium, creatinine and urea but also daily measures of magnesium and phosphate to guard against refeeding dangers (see Chapter 8). Measurements are also needed before IVN is commenced in order to provide baseline results that help to determine appropriate additions to the initial bag. Ideally measurements for several days before IVN should be taken into account to identify any trends in renal function. Daily measures are usually required for at least the first 1–2 weeks of IVN until patients become stable enough to decrease the frequency of assessment. Calcium levels, corrected for albumin, need to be checked twice weekly during early IVN, with more frequent assessment in patients with renal impairment or those with abnormal levels.

Monitoring liver function

Interpreting laboratory liver function tests must take into account the pattern as well as the level of abnormality. Liver problems are often either predominantly due to hepatocellular dysfunction, with a hepatitic pattern of changes in the tests, or predominantly due to biliary dysfunction or obstruction, with a cholestatic pattern of change. A typical hepatitic picture would be a normal or low albumin, a definitely raised alanine or aspartate transferase (ALT or AST) and a normal or raised bilirubin and alkaline phosphatase (ALP). A typical cholestatic picture would be a definitely raised bilirubin and/or ALP with less raised or normal ALT or AST. These 'typical' patterns are sometimes misleading, however, and the picture in established cirrhosis due to either cholestatic or hepatitic processes can be very confusing. Indeed, it can be easy to miss the diagnosis of significant chronic liver disease since a shrunken scarred organ may no longer have the cell mass to produce high levels of liver enzymes. These can therefore be normal or low, even with ongoing inflammation or obstruction, and although bilirubin levels may be raised, this is not inevitable. The only laboratory abnormalities in liver cirrhosis can therefore be a raised international normalised ratio (INR) and/or low albumin due to poor liver synthetic function, with additional clues coming from a low platelet count (due to the hypersplenism of portal hypertension and poor bone marrow function). A low sodium may also occur due to the propensity for liver patients to retain relatively more water than salt, even though the total body content of both is actually high (see Chapter 10).

As with electrolytes and renal function, it is useful to measure baseline levels of liver function prior to commencing IVN. Repeat measures are then needed about twice weekly until the patient is stable. Failure of the liver to clear lipid from the blood can result in laboratory reports of lipaemic blood samples, although if this occurs you should first check that the sample was not taken from the catheter with IVN running, which causes contamination with IVN (see Chapter 8). IVN lipids contain triglycerides (see Chapter 7) so it may be useful to monitor lipid profiles in some patients, e.g. those with known hyperlipidaemia.

If abnormalities of liver function develop in an IVN patient, they are often due to problems other than the IVN itself (see Chapter 12). However, if this is not the case and the IVN is thought to be responsible, changes in the regimen will be needed, as discussed in Chapter 12.

Monitoring micronutrients and trace elements

Measurements of micronutrient and trace element levels are expensive and time-consuming. Many of the levels are also influenced by the acute-phase response, e.g. zinc levels fall in acute illness with the fall in albumin[3] and vitamin A levels fall with a decline in retinol-binding protein[4]. Acute measurement of micronutrient status is not therefore indicated unless there is a specific reason to do so, as long as you are giving appropriate micronutrients in the IVN (see Chapter 9).

Monitoring issues in long-term IVN patients

Many of the monitoring recommendations for long-term IVN and home IVN patients are the same as for short-term patients, but at much reduced intervals. However, some aspects of their review do differ in terms of both clinical and laboratory assessment and some complications occur in long-term IVN use that are not generally seen in shorter-term patients.

Routine clinical review

As with any IVN patient, assessment of general appearance and well-being is important. You should particularly look for evidence of specific deficiencies or excesses caused by the long-term administration of regimens containing incorrect levels of micronutrients (see Chapter 9). Changes in body weight are critical in determining whether you are providing adequate but not excessive energy, but it is important that any apparent weight change takes into account possible changes in fluid balance. Results vary considerably depending on when weight is recorded in relation to the time of day when IVN is used and the day of the week for patients who do not feed on every day.

Questions should be asked about any infective symptoms such as fevers, rigors, sweating or malaise to identify any possible problems. However, even in the absence of such symptoms, you must consider the possibility of 'grumbling' infection that might 'seed' to the intravenous catheter or progress in its own right.

Laboratory review

A review of recent laboratory results is important to look for both acute problems and trends. Checking liver function is particularly important in view of the potential for IVN to cause long-term liver damage (see Chapter 12). Review is needed at least 3-monthly in stable patients and you must be aware that slow damage may lead to cirrhosis, with very little in the way of clinical or laboratory abnormalities until 90% or more of the organ function is lost (see above). A high index of suspicion is needed to differentiate between possible IVN-induced liver dysfunction and damage from other potential sources (see Chapter 12).

In the longer-term IVN patient, monitoring of vitamin and trace element status is also important. We usually check micronutrients levels at 3- or 6-month intervals once the patient is stable. High manganese levels, which can cause basal ganglia damage and movement disorders are relatively common in this cohort of patients, although problems of both deficiency and toxicity can occur following prolonged IVN use (see Chapter 9).

Bone density

Specific consideration of bone density is required for patients who are on long-term IVN. Both osteoporosis and osteomalacia can occur and baseline dual-spectrum X-ray densitometry (DEXA) scanning should be performed on all new home IVN patients once they are stable. It should then be repeated at 2-yearly intervals or more frequently if problems are developing. Some patients, especially those with short-bowel syndrome, will require regular bisphosphanate, usually given parenterally every 3 months. Checking of parathyroid hormone, 1, 25-dihydroxyvitamin D and 25-hydroxyvitamin D levels is also advised.

References

1. NICE and the National Collaborating Centre For Acute Care. *Nutrition Support in Adults: Oral Nutrition Support, Enteral Tube Feeding and Parenteral Nutrition*. London: NICE and the National Collaborating Centre For Acute Care, 2006.
2. Davies D, Ferner R, Glanville H, eds. *Davies's Textbook of Adverse Drug Reactions*, 5th edn. London: Chapman and Hall, 1998: 459–460.
3. Payne-James, Grimble G, Silk D, eds. *Artificial Nutrition Support in Clinical Practice*, 2nd edn. London: Greenwich Medical Media, 2001: 204–205.
4. Payne-James, Grimble G, Silk D, eds. *Artificial Nutrition Support in Clinical Practice*, 2nd edn. London: Greenwich Medical Media, 2001: 200–201.

14

Organising nutrition support

Introduction

Providing adequate nutrition to all patients should be one of the aims of all hospitals. In most cases, patients' needs will be met by the catering services but in some, nutrition support by oral, enteral tube feeding or intravenous nutrition (IVN) will be required. Those prescribing IVN should therefore work within this broader context, ideally practising in an appropriately structured nutrition support team (NST) which works alongside dietitians, nurses and caterers to deliver overall nutritional care. Details of the organisation and funding to ensure such arrangements are too complex to cover in detail in this book but nevertheless, all IVN prescribers should have a broad understanding of:

- The organisation of all local nutrition services
- Different types of NST
- The structure of an NST
- The role of an active NST
- Individual responsibilities within an NST
- Funding opportunities for NSTs
- Local IVN purchasing arrangements (see Chapter 15)

Organisation of local nutrition services

The provision of adequate nutrition for all involves many diverse services which are not necessarily accountable to those with responsibility for nutrition policy. Hospitals should therefore have a system to bring together catering managers, senior nurses, pharmacists, dietitians and clinicians, to ensure that sensible, cost-effective policies are pursued. The National Institute for Health and Clinical Excellence (NICE) recommends that all hospitals should have a nutrition steering committee[1] for this purpose and that all IVN prescribing should be undertaken and monitored by a multidisciplinary NST. The British Association for Parenteral and Enteral Nutrition also recommends

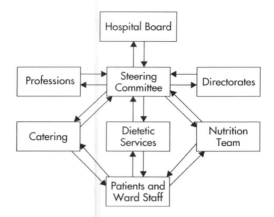

Figure 14.1 Structure of nutrition support.

setting up nutrition steering committees and NSTs[2], suggesting that the former should comprise at least:

- A business manager accountable to the chief executive of the hospital
- The lead nutrition team consultant
- The chief pharmacist
- The chief dietitian
- The director of nursing
- The chief catering officer
- A specialist nutrition nurse

This steering committee should take overall responsibility for a variety of issues within local nutritional management, including some aspects of practice and policy in routine catering, oral supplementation, enteral tube feeding and IVN. Their decisions can then be implemented within the framework shown in Figure 14.1.

Different types of nutrition support team

As shown in Figure 14.1, the nutrition steering committee oversees the activities of the hospital NST. However, there are wide differences in the day-to-day operations of NSTs which vary with local skills, interest and funding. Most hospitals that have an NST use one of three models:

1. The strategic model
2. The supervisory model
3. The active patient management model

The strategic nutrition support team

In this arrangement, the NST operates at a distance from patients and is not directly involved in their care. The team usually contains dietitians, nurses, pharmacists and clinicians but their only aim as a team is to discuss the needs of the local nutrition service and to set standards for nutritional care. They do not usually discuss the needs of specific patients. As such, they really attempt to undertake the business of a nutrition steering committee but frequently lack the seniority or breadth of representation to allow them to do so effectively. This approach also offers little support to the health care professionals responsible for the routine nutritional management of patients and may lead to health care professionals with limited practical experience of IVN are advising on its use.

We would not recommend this model and it does not comply with NICE guidelines.

The supervisory nutrition support team

In this arrangement, specialists with an interest in nutrition get together to discuss the nutritional management of specific patients. This usually occurs once a week or less frequently and patient discussions are generally office-based, case note reviews rather than bedside assessments. This approach allows joint team decisions and to some extent staff can learn from each other's different expertise. Nevertheless, it does not permit a true multidisciplinary review of patients as their needs arise and it does not give the NST any presence on the wards. As a consequence, the team has less influence and there is far from ideal liaison and co-ordination with other clinical teams.

The active patient management nutrition support team

Active patient management should be the aim of all NSTs supervising patients on IVN. This approach involves team rounds on all weekdays to review all IVN patients. The core nutrition team assesses referrals, prescribes IVN where indicated and advises on the suitability of intravenous access, electrolyte management, fluid provision and alternatives to IVN use. In many cases the NST is also involved in complex oral or enterally supported patients, especially the placement and management of enteral feeding tubes including gastrostomies. This model brings expertise to each patient and hence should minimise incorrect IVN use and consequent costly complications. The presence of the NST on the wards allows close liaison and numerous educational opportunities to make sure that all clinical staff understand the risks and benefits of IVN usage.

The structure of an active nutrition support team

The core NST is usually made up of professionals responsible for the day-to-day nutritional management of patients on IVN whereas dietitians usually manage patients on oral nutrition support and deal with most aspects of enteral tube feeding. It is essential to have an appropriate skill mix in the core NST, which ideally should include at least one full-time nutrition nurse specialist along with significant funded input from at least one pharmacist and one dietitian who have particular interests in nutrition support.

The NST should also be able to access on a daily basis a clinician who is fully trained in clinical nutrition and it is also valuable to have more junior clinician involvement, e.g. a specialist registrar who assists in service provision while receiving training in clinical nutrition support. Consultant and trainee gastroenterologists are the most common clinicians to contribute to NSTs but there are also many general surgeons, anaesthetists, intensivists and chemical pathologists involved.

The nursing, dietetic and pharmacist members of the nutrition team should be appointed at appropriate grades to reflect the specialist knowledge, skills and experience required. The whole-time equivalents of each team member will be determined by a variety of local factors, particularly the workload in different aspects of local NST function. These factors include:

- *Usual inpatient IVN-related workload*: this includes initial assessments, daily reviews, prescribing when appropriate and provision of advice as IVN finishes and patients move on to oral or enteral tube nutrition.
- *Need for specialist advice for non-IVN nutrition patients*: this includes issues such as appropriate management of fluid and electrolytes in short-bowel patients, refeeding problems in severe anorexia nervosa patients and problems with placement and maintenance of enteral feeding tubes.
- *Home IVN patient-related workload*: this includes regular outpatient clinical review, monitoring and prescription along with

commitments related to their admissions for complications such as catheter-related sepsis.

- *Other NST services provided locally*: such as review of the referrals for percutaneous endosopic gastrostomy placement.
- *Clinical records, data management and audit.*
- *Education and training commitments.*

The time required for an effective service in the areas above should not be underestimated. An initial IVN patient assessment may require up to 60 minutes and daily review (with prescribing when necessary) often takes 20–30 minutes, especially as there are inevitable delays such as unavailable patients or ward clinicians tied up elsewhere. You must also include all aspects of service provision, not just bedside activities. For example, the need to look up reported biochemistry and to collect and audit data is also very time-consuming. Furthermore, team members may have significant commitments elsewhere, e.g. pharmacist time within other pharmaceutical services such as Technical Services.

If only one person can be permanently allocated to a nutrition team, it should be a clinical nurse specialist, recognising that there will still be a need for regular pharmacy and dietetic input. This is in keeping with the NICE recommendations[1] and reflects the need for practical nursing skills in reducing risks from intravenous catheters (especially catheter-related sepsis) and enteral tube access.

Roles within an active nutrition support team

As mentioned throughout this book, the main role of most hospital nutrition teams is to assess, review and monitor patients requiring IVN and to ensure that they receive correctly prescribed regimens by either prescribing them themselves or supervising the prescription of others (although the latter is not ideal – see below).

Although different team members have different skills, it is possible for their roles to overlap significantly and this will increase team efficiency. For example, although some teams operate policies whereby a new referral is seen separately by a nurse, dietitian, pharmacist and clinician, an experienced professional from any one of the above groups should be capable of making an initial assessment in most patients, deciding on whether IVN is appropriate and determining the regimen that is needed. They should also be able to identify all types of IVN-related problems and so daily ward rounds can be made by any one or more of nurse specialist, pharmacist, dietitian or NST clinician.

However, when patient reviews are undertaken without the full team, efforts must be made to update the other team members so that they remain familiar with developments in all current IVN patients and know about all new referrals. The updates will also ensure that individual expertise is used to solve any potential difficulties and to check that no mistakes are being made. Input from the NST clinicians should ideally be on ward rounds carried out at least once or twice weekly, with further informal availability to discuss or see patients at other times.

Using overlapping roles as outlined above also projects an image of a professional team and allows immediate cover for annual leave and sickness. In addition, it also offers professional development opportunities and ensures that every team member has the knowledge and experience to recognise when cases are complicated and hence when multidisciplinary input is required. Team members who take part in this type of role overlap should not feel that they are losing control of their specialist area but instead should recognise that they gain additional skills and responsibilities.

The potential for overlapping roles in NSTs is shown in Figure 14.2.

In addition to their shared roles, each NST member has jobs which are more specific in terms of their expertise. These jobs include:

- *Specialist nutrition nurses*: extensive involvement in central line care and especially measures to ensure aseptic handling of IVN catheters by other nursing and medical staff.
- *NST pharmacist*: consideration of local medicines formulary, the potential reuse of IVN bags when appropriate (see Chapter 15) and support to the pharmacy department and Technical Services. Monitoring of, reporting on and taking steps to control IVN-related expenditure are common additional roles for the NST pharmacist.
- *NST dietitian*: close involvement with patients who are fed using a combination of IVN and oral/enteral methods and supervision of patients stopping IVN in order to ensure that they maintain an adequate nutrient intake.

It has been suggested that specialist active NSTs 'de-skill' other health care professionals because they lose the opportunity to be involved in the nutritional management of some more complex patients. This can be true but a good NST should also offer opportunities to staff with an interest. These opportunities include:

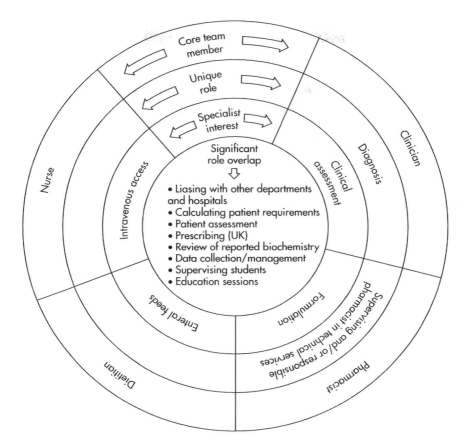

Figure 14.2 Examples of role overlap in the core nutrition team.

- *Formal nutrition teaching sessions*: for a wide variety of health care professionals and students (the different professions in the team can offer different learning perspectives).
- *Chances to join specialist NST ward rounds*: these provide ideal learning opportunities for any interested professional or student.
- *Specialist advice*: for other health care professionals responsible for the patient.
- *Other informal teaching opportunities*: for staff on wards or in clinics.

A dedicated active NST will ensure that the risks of IVN are minimised and can also remove the burden of complex IVN prescribing from the workload of others. In the past this always involved advising on the prescription which then needed to be written or at least signed by a doctor. In recent times this has changed in the UK with the introduction of supplementary prescribing and more recently still by changes that allow independent prescribing of IVN by suitably expert nurses and pharmacists.

Supplementary and independent prescribing (UK)

Supplementary prescribing is a form of non-clinician prescribing introduced into the UK with the Health and Social Care Act 2001. It allows various health care professionals to prescribe legally and take the appropriate responsibility for their decisions[3]. Before registering as supplementary prescribers with their professional body, health care professionals must successfully complete an approved university course under the direction of a local clinician mentor of consultant level. The course content varies between institutions but generally includes:

- *Set taught sessions*: including lectures, distance-learning study and practical skills sessions
- *Practice journal*: evidence of time spent with the mentor to learn about prescribing issues and to prove competence
- *Examinations*

Once registered, supplementary prescribing must be incorporated into job descriptions to ensure vicarious liability. Once a clinician has made a diagnosis for a patient, supplementary prescribing can be used in that patient subject to patient consent and the consent of both the clinician (the independent prescriber) and the supplementary prescriber. A clinical management plan must also be put in the patient's case notes, detailing what can and cannot be prescribed by the supplementary prescriber and adding any specific conditions. The clinical management plan can be either restrictive or allow a considerable degree of prescribing freedom. In the case of IVN it is logical to allow for any regimen design since the needs within one patient can vary widely but the supplementary prescriber must always act within his or her competence and must seek advice from the independent prescriber if at all unsure. It is therefore essential to have ready access to the independent prescriber.

The process of supplementary prescribing allows a legal overlap between other NST specialists and the traditional clinician role. The benefits include:

- Cost savings for the same level of prescribing competence compared to a clinician

- Decreased commitments for independent prescribers to permit more time with patients who need their clinical input
- Ready access to the prescriber for Technical Services (see Chapter 15) in the case of any queries
- A more professional NST with the high level of knowledge and skill required to prescribe safely and appropriately

At the time of writing (2006), further changes to UK law have just been introduced which permit non-clinician, independent prescribing for nurses and pharmacists. These changes will undoubtedly be adopted by some NSTs to enhance their multidisciplinary effectiveness.

The expanded nutrition team

The core members of an NST cannot work in isolation and must rely on others to provide the complete daily nutrition service. All others involved should be encouraged to think of themselves as part of an expanded nutrition team which incorporates a wide variety of staff, including:

- *Ward pharmacists*: to exchange ideas on the general drug and nutritional management of patients.
- *Ward nurses*: who administer the IVN and have a role in monitoring for some complications, e.g. temperature.
- *Ward clinicians*: who are responsible for the patient and determine if the patient is permitted oral or enteral tube intake.
- *Diabetes team*: for help with the management of complex patients with persistent hypo- or hyperglycaemia. Often helpful with diabetic patients moving to cyclical IVN over less than 24 hours (see Chapter 7).
- *Microbiology*: to provide specialist advice relating to the management of catheter-related sepsis.
- *Chemical pathology/biochemistry*: to report laboratory results, to provide advice on the interpretation of complex results, to recommend appropriate tests in complex clinical cases.
- *Dietetics*: to provide advice on oral or enteral feeding, more specialist products, and special nutritional needs.
- *Technical Services*: to provide advice on IVN formulation and stability and, locally, to compound (or order in) the prescribed IVN regimens.
- *Logistics*: to ensure an appropriate continued supply of products and for help with contracting issues.

- *Home nutrition company*: who formulate, compound and offer some trouble-shooting of patients requiring home IVN.

One of the benefits of a multidisciplinary core nutrition team is that the individual specialist members can liaise as appropriate with their equivalents within the expanded team. This leads to greater influence when trying to ensure that the importance of nutritional care moves up the agenda for all health professionals even if they have no direct responsibility for nutrition support.

Data collection, management and review

NSTs need to know what they are doing and (for reasons of clinical governance, audit, research and financial planning) whether they are doing it safely and effectively. A good team must therefore record data on:

- How many patients they are asked to see, where they are and what is wrong with them
- How many of these patients start IVN and for how long they receive it
- Whether IVN was stopped because it was no longer needed or because of an IVN-related complication
- The nature of all IVN complications
- How many patients the NST sees who receive other means of nutrition support, i.e. all NST activities related to enteral tube feeding or orally supported patients, including requests related to enteral tube placement or blockage and activities such as assessment for percutaneous endoscopic gastrostomies (PEGs)
- Any other activities such as education and training

The aims and nature of data collection

The reasons for data collection are numerous and vary with local needs. They generally include:

- *Evidence of good practice*: you need to know whether the overall complication rates that you see with IVN usage are reasonable compared to those reported from other centres and whether there are variations in rates between different ward areas, suggesting either particularly good or bad practice from which lessons may be learned; procedures changed/implemented or education provided.

- *Evidence of NST workload*: any discussions on funding either informally or within formal business developments need evidence of the amount and type of work undertaken by the NST. Costs and potential cost savings can then be calculated (see below). Data need to be collected over prolonged periods (i.e. several years) to ensure that apparent trends do not simply reflect natural variations in patient numbers.
- *Data for research purposes*: many NSTs conduct clinically oriented research which requires records of changes in outcome with changes in the type or nature of intervention.

Always be clear from the outset why particular information should be collected and regularly review whether the data you record remain relevant. A data collection form will be needed and the whole form must be filled in so that subsequent entry on to a computer database is as simple and consistent as possible. Be clear about all entries on the form so that no subsequent interpretation is required. Table 14.1 shows examples of the data that are likely to be useful.

Data storage and management

Gathering data is of no value unless it can be stored and analysed efficiently. This will require the use of a computer database but care is needed since:

- The Data Protection Act will apply in the UK (register databases locally)
- There is a risk of data loss

Records should be kept up to date and permit easy access to the information you are likely to need. The type of software that you use (e.g. Microsoft Excel or Microsoft Access) will be dictated by local knowledge, skills and support. Do not underestimate the time required for appropriate data management, especially entry of any back-data if information that was not initially included in the database has to be extracted from patients' notes or team records.

In all cases, data must be as simple and consistent as possible. For example, do not include both 'postoperative ileus' and 'post-op ileus' but choose one way of expressing the indication. This will make interpretation accurate and simpler. Once you have extracted the data

Table 14.1 Basic nutrition team data collection form

Section	Data	Reason for collection	Comments
Referrals	Data log number	To describe total data collection	Allows cross-referencing to original paper copies of data collected
Patient identifiers and referral patterns	Day of referral	For trend analysis	For example, are there many requests for IVN on Friday afternoons or on days when nutrition team clinicians attend ward rounds?
	Year and month of referral	For filtering of data	During data processing you need to be able to define activity during different periods
	Ward and directorate	To identify where the patient was based	To identify nutrition team workloads and to filter patients by area
	Patient group	To allow subgrouping of patients within directorates	Particularly useful for business cases. Examples would include 'oesophagogastric', 'hepatobiliary', 'pancreatic', 'colorectal' and 'urological' groups within General Surgery or 'bone marrow transplant' or 'non-transplant' within Haemato-oncology
	Age	For describing your IVN population	
	Primary diagnosis	Description of patient population	Be accurate and consistent
	Reason for referral	Data are needed on numbers of patients referred for IVN versus numbers referred, e.g. for enteral tube problems	All activities need to be recorded since they contribute to the nutrition team workload

Table 14.1 Continued

Section	Data	Reason for collection	Comments
	Days postoperation	To describe your local population and referral practices by the various ward teams/consultants	
Nutritional state	Weight loss	To monitor referrals for IVN	Required for MUST scoring
	Body mass index	For describing your IVN population	Required for MUST scoring
	Days no effective nutrition	To review whether local nutritional care plans are implemented and are appropriate. To evaluate how long teams wait before referring for IVN	Use precise data if possible, e.g. 'days of inadequate nutrition on review' or 'duration of IVN' should not say '>14' if at all possible because this will mean the data interpretation will not be accurate. Always use precise numbers if possible. Required for MUST scoring
	Screening tool score, e.g. MUST	For describing your local IVN population	Can be used to determine how effectively local nutritional care plans are implemented following routine nutritional screening
	Oedema score on referral	Excessive salt and water provision can cause or delay return of gastrointestinal function	To indicate whether fluid management problems may have contributed to intestinal dysfunction

(cont.)

Table 14.1 Continued

Section	Data	Reason for collection	Comments
Intravenous access	Intravenous access	Type of access may be related to complication rates and has resource implications	Depending on local workload and practices, you may be interested in comparing peripheral against central intravenous access for the use of IVN or the number of lumens of a central line against the likelihood of line sepsis. Also for reporting line sepsis rates
IVN usage	Indication for IVN	Description of why IVN is being used	This needs to be as specific as possible. For example, 'poor nutritional status' should not be entered as the indication for IVN since it tells you little of use and, similarly, 'complicated surgery and 20 days no nutrition' is also too vague since there may be many reasons for restricting nutritional intake via the gut following surgery (e.g. 'prolonged postoperative ileus', 'concerns regarding anastomotic integrity', 'no gastrointestinal access for nutrition support')
	Outcome of referral	The type of nutrition support provided	Identifies patients who were not considered suitable for IVN and is therefore an important parameter for cost savings analysis
	Days of IVN	Essential information when assessing complication rates	Directly relevant to nutrition team patient costs

Table 14.1 Continued

Section	Data	Reason for collection	Comments
	Number of bags of IVN	Direct relation to workload and IVN-related costs	Not the same as days of IVN, since some bags may be run over more than 24 hours (see Chapters 7 and 11)
	Reason IVN stopped	To determine whether the patient progressed or a complication occurred, e.g. loss of intravenous access or catheter-related sepsis. This should be the primary reason that IVN was discontinued. Provides evidence that particular patients receiving IVN were appropriately given it but were forced to stop as a result of a complication	Once again, accuracy is important, e.g. if the patient was on half-rate IVN and planned to stop the following day due to progress to oral diet but became septic that following day. This could be interpreted as either 'progress to oral diet' or 'suspected sepsis' but the former is correct because the IVN would have been discontinued anyway. If the IVN would have been continued then 'suspected sepsis' is the more appropriate option. Do not include both as this would complicate data interpretation and make filtering difficult
Patient outcome	Outcome following IVN	Such as 'progress to diet' or 'enteral tube feeding', 'withdrawal of treatment', 'death'	
Non-clinician prescribing	Non-clinician prescribing	Such as 'supplementary prescribing' in the UK to demonstrate both time and financial savings by the nutrition team and to demonstrate the effectiveness of local prescribing systems	

(cont.)

Table 14.1 Continued

Section	Data	Reason for collection	Comments
Complications	Complications of IVN	To demonstrate where local practice may need improvement, e.g. lack of biochemistry monitoring, inappropriate access of intravenous catheters. To provide a record of local complication rates to benchmark against other centres	

IVN, intravenous nutrition; MUST, Malnutrition Universal Screening Tool[4].

that you require it should be interpreted in context, e.g. new services increasing workload. Always provide the time period to which your presented data relate – e.g. whether it is the financial year or the calendar year – to aid matching to data from other sources.

Funding opportunities for nutrition support teams

Many hospitals either have no NST or a team with only one funded member of staff. You may therefore need to construct a business case to allow the establishment or expansion of a team. Funding may be based on a variety of mechanisms, including:

- *Limiting inappropriate IVN use*: most NSTs should find that they can avoid the use of IVN in up to 25% of referrals. This amounts to very substantial annual cost savings.
- *Avoiding IVN-related complications*: the cost of a single episode of catheter-related sepsis has been put at up to £5000 in 1992[5], since each episode is likely to prolong hospital stay and require the use of expensive intravenous drugs. Studies have shown that the presence of NSTs reduces catheter-related sepsis rates, in some cases from levels of 30% or more to single-percentage figures. It therefore seems likely that the presence of an active NST will save at least one expensive episode of catheter-related sepsis for every 10 patients put on to IVN. This means that savings should amount to well over £100 000 annually in most large hospitals where IVN is used appropriately.
- *Avoiding bag wastage*: utilising bags compounded for one patient but not given (e.g. because of catheter-related sepsis, loss of access, improved gastrointestinal function: see Chapter 15) is only possible when a single team is aware of all IVN patients' needs and so can redirect that bag to another suitable recipient.
- *Saving clinicians' time*: NST members are generally paid significantly less than clinicians who would otherwise have to spend long periods assessing, reviewing and prescribing for IVN referrals (an important point in the context of the European Working Time Directive and the consequent need to reduce doctors' hours[6]).
- *Provision of specific services*: NST activities related to enteral feeding tubes can also save complications and costs. For example, screening all referrals for gastrostomy to ensure that they are appropriate and safe, and to determine whether they are best

placed endoscopically or radiologically, generates huge savings through avoiding pointless procedures and reducing wasted slots in endoscopy and the X-ray department (not to mention putting patients through inappropriate procedures, which may result in significant distress for both them and their family).

- *Education and training sessions*: it is usually possible to identify direct local savings as well as less easily costed savings through reduced IVN and enteral feeding tube complications when the workforce has been properly trained. An example would be the reduction in unnecessary chest X-rays to check nasogastric tube position if the nutrition nurse trains staff to place and check tubes correctly. Teaching activities can also bring in external income, e.g. from training days.
- *Professional time in non-NST roles*: a primarily nutrition team role may be supported by funding for time in another role.

Funding models

In view of the above, nutrition teams should aim to maintain clear records of their activity to identify all potential funding streams. Funding for the nutrition team for the review, management and prescribing (where appropriate) of hospital inpatients can be obtained from one of three main methods:

1. *'Top-slicing'*: a fixed amount is taken from users of the service at the beginning of the financial year. This has the huge advantage of immediately ensuring team funding for the year, allowing them to concentrate on patient care and developments. The level of funding may be determined by the workload of each user (e.g. for 'surgery' or 'medicine'), although this may be variable resulting in compli-cations.

2. *From each type of NST service*: which may be many and varied, e.g. income from teaching, funding for research, cost savings from non-use of IVN, cost savings from enteral feeding services and assessment of patients for gastrostomy (see above). Some sources of this funding may be variable but the model can avoid 'unfunded' but regular input into other local services.

3. *'Cost per bag'*: an 'on-cost' is added to the cost of each bag prescribed. This income may be variable, may not account for the time spent on non-prescribing activities, could present a conflict of interests and is likely to be added to a drugs budget rather than a staffing budget. If properly managed, however, this can be simple

and it allows users to pay for the service as they require it. It also allows for automatically funded increases in workload.

More than one of the above approaches may be necessary and it is important to ensure funding is used for its intended purpose. Regular review is required to avoid unfunded significant additional work, which is determined by referrals and not by the nutrition team. The nutrition team determines which of those referrals it receives actually require IVN (see above).

There are some arguments for the nutrition team holding its own budget as it keeps things clearer and there are fewer complications than when income is kept within others' budgets. Funds should be allocated for aspects including salaries, equipment and training but should probably not be held for drugs (including the cost of the IVN) to avoid conflicts of interest. Although responsibility for the IVN cost should lie with those referring the patients, providing advice on expenditure and reduction in drug costs, e.g. managing the appropriate reuse of unused bags, is an important role of the nutrition team (see above).

References

1.   NICE and the National Collaborating Centre For Acute Care. *Nutrition Support in Adults: Oral Nutrition Support, Enteral Tube Feeding and Parenteral Nutrition*. London: NICE and the National Collaborating Centre For Acute Care, 2006.
2.   Pennington C, ed. *Current Perspectives on Parenteral Nutrition in Adults: A Report by a Working Party of the British Association for Parenteral and Enteral Nutrition*. Maidenhead: British Association of Parenteral and Enteral Nutrition, 1996: 13–15.
3.   Bellingham C. How supplementary prescribing helps in both acute and chronic hospital care. *Pharm J* 2004; 272: 640–641.
4.   Malnutrition Advisory Group. http://www.bapen.org.uk/the-must.htm (accessed 13 June 2006).
5.   Lennard-Jones J, ed. *A Positive Approach to Nutrition as Treatment*. London: King's Fund, 1992.
6.   Department of Health. *Protecting Staff; Delivering Services Implementing the European Working Time Directive for Doctors in Training*. Health Service circular HSC 2003/001. London: Department of Health, 2003.

15

Technical Services

Introduction

One of the most important elements in providing safe and effective intravenous nutrition (IVN) at minimum cost are Technical Services, who compound the prescribed IVN regimens and manage much of the logistics related to all aspects of IVN supply. Technical Services usually refers to a dedicated section within the hospital pharmacy but may also refer to an external compounding unit. Compounding facilities are sometimes called by other local names depending on preferences, e.g. 'aseptics' or 'pharmacy production'.

Technical Services are an integral part of the prescribing process (Figure 15.1) since the prescriber must work with the unit to ensure that a suitable, stable regimen is provided to all patients within a reasonable timeframe. Negotiation is also required on the products which should be stocked and those that should be ordered on specific request. Figure 15.1 shows some of the many jobs undertaken by Technical Services following receipt of an IVN prescription.

Why compound intravenous nutrition regimens in Technical Services?

Compounding IVN is complex and often requires many separate additions to each bag. With such a complex mixture of components there is a high potential for instability, compounding errors and the inclusion of contaminants and infective agents.

Regimen stability

There are three types of IVN stability that need to be controlled to ensure the safety of the patient (Box 15.1). All prescribers of IVN regimens must be aware of the physical and chemical stability of each bag they prescribe. Although a check of these aspects is carried out within

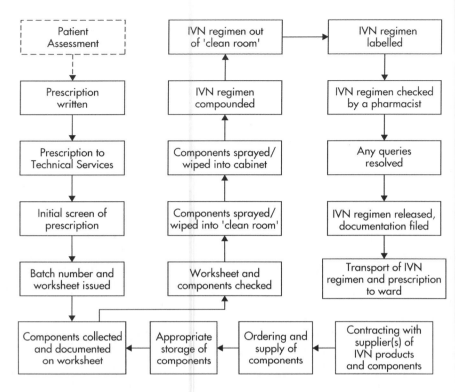

Figure 15.1 Example of processes involved in arranging an intravenous nutrition regimen following prescribing (subject to local variations).

Technical Services before the compounded bag is released (see below), this check should not be relied upon as the prescriber has direct responsibility. Appendix 1 contains some details about physical and chemical stability but if questions arise you should always seek advice from your local Technical Services.

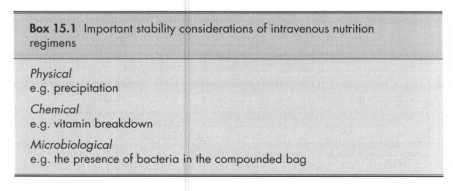

Box 15.1 Important stability considerations of intravenous nutrition regimens

Physical
e.g. precipitation

Chemical
e.g. vitamin breakdown

Microbiological
e.g. the presence of bacteria in the compounded bag

The microbiological stability of a regimen is controlled within Technical Services by using cabinets within special rooms called 'clean rooms' (Plate 5). These, with a number of additional controls, minimise the risk of contaminating the bag during compounding. It is the 'critical zone' within the cabinet where compounding actually takes place. Cabinets and clean rooms vary in design but all must meet strict standards as part of comprehensive local quality assurance systems that are in place to ensure the safety of the patient. Regular monitoring of the background contamination in the clean room is mandatory.

Contamination of IVN regimens during compounding has proved fatal[1]. Compounded IVN is an ideal microbiological growth medium and, if contamination occurs, the rapidly multiplying micro-organisms are given to patients by direct intravenous infusion which bypasses many natural defences. All IVN regimens must therefore be compounded inside controlled and managed units where the risks to the patient are appropriately minimised. This includes making additions to any IVN bag (even if physical and chemical stability are known) as well as changing a giving set that has already been fitted (see Chapter 16 and Appendix 1). Fitting a giving set to an IVN bag which does not already have one fitted, can be undertaken in a clinical environment rather than a specialised unit if absolutely necessary but the practice should be discouraged and strict aseptic technique must be used. More details on aseptic compounding facilities and techniques are given in Appendix 1.

Compounding technique and accuracy

All operators compounding IVN bags for patients must be validated to ensure their aseptic technique is of the required standard for the facilities within which they work, i.e they must be consistently accurate in the clean facilities available locally. The aseptic technique they use must also minimise the risk of final product contamination (Box 15.2). All operators are therefore highly trained and regularly assessed (Appendix 1).

Documentation

Comprehensive documentation of all compounding processes is required following the basic rule that 'if it is not documented, it did not happen'. For this reason, appropriately designed documentation must be completed at every step to provide evidence of what was done by whom. All documentation should be archived in case it is required in the future, e.g. component or packaging recall.

Box 15.2 Potential contaminants of intravenous nutrition (IVN) bags during compounding

Viable
e.g. bacteria and fungi

Non-viable
e.g. particulates

Chemical
e.g. cross-contamination between products

Note: viruses are obligate intracellular parasites and are therefore not considered a practical risk to compounded IVN bags

---

Unit documentation must also include validated 'standard process instructions' or 'standard operating procedures' that detail exactly how a process is to be carried out each time with no room for interpretation. This ensures one result from the same process to permit close monitoring and compounding accuracy.

Final bag release

The final release of a compounded IVN regimen requires an understanding of the whole Technical Services unit as well as the principles and standards that determine its operation. This process is carried out by a trained and locally approved pharmacist (subject to locally applicable regulations).

It is usual practice for a pharmacist to screen IVN prescriptions to detect obvious prescribing errors and to ensure the relevance of bag additions. There are, however, limitations to this screening process. A standard prescription administered to a patient retaining electrolytes due to severe acute renal failure could be fatal but whether this would be picked up would depend on the level of detail of the local screening process.

When pharmaceutically checking any item, it is important to be logical and to follow a set pattern. All aspects must be covered each time in order to ensure that nothing has been missed (Box 15.3). Everything should be related to the primary document (i.e. the prescription) because of the risk of transcription errors.

Appropriate resolution of any anomalies detected is necessary but their significance varies and as not all will warrant discarding the bag. This means that, as an IVN prescriber, you may be contacted if an error

---

Box 15.3 Example of the final release of compounded intravenous nutrition regimens

---

1 Identify product(s) and documentation, including batch number on each – if there is any doubt that they relate to each other then recompounding is necessary
2 Confirm prescription as being clinically appropriate (subject to local limitations)
3 Confirm correct transcription of prescription on to the worksheet
4 Confirm number of ingredients on all worksheets is correct (if more than one worksheet)
5 Check all worksheet calculations
6 Check that the formula resulting from the calculations meets the prescription requirements
7 Check all worksheet check-signatures are present
8 Confirm the stability of the formula
9 Check each product and label for patient details, dispensed item number, day of use, nutritional levels, electrolyte and additive levels, total volume, expiry date and whether the bag may be administered either peripherally or centrally or if it should only be administered centrally
10 Check the number of bags present matches the number requested on the worksheet and all labels printed are accounted for
11 Check the identity of premixed bag (if used)
12 Check all clamps and air vents to ensure that they are closed, and end-cap on giving-set (if applicable) to ensure that it is in place
13 Check each bag for leaks, the presence of additive-port cap and particles (precipitation, 'coring' and scratch threads of plastic)
14 Identify that packaging, products are sealed and dispatched correctly

Note: Any pharmacist release checking must understand all of the general principles and standards of Technical Services as well as the local systems in place (which is beyond the remit of this book).

---

has been detected but the bag may still be appropriate for the patient, e.g. a total sodium of 210 mmol rather than 200 mmol is likely to be usable for the same patient whereas a total potassium of 20 mmol rather than 0 mmol probably cannot be used (see Chapters 8 and 10). If there is any doubt over the suitability of the compounded bag it should always be discarded and recompounded or a decision made to wait until the next day to continue IVN.

All errors warrant discussion with the staff involved to determine the cause, to review the relevant quality assurance systems and to ensure that the error is not repeated. Carelessness or taking short cuts is always unacceptable and should be treated very seriously.

A visual inspection of the product is an important aspect of the final release process (Box 15.3). Whilst subtle problems may be more easily detected using techniques such as theoretical stability tables, a visual inspection can show obvious errors. Plate 6a shows the normal appearance of a lipid-containing IVN regimen, whereas the bag on the left of Plate 6b shows a lipid-free regimen (the yellow colour is due to the nitrogen/vitamin component used). It should be immediately obvious to a trained pharmacist that the bag to the right of Plate 6b is a compounding error as it resembles neither a normal lipid nor lipid-free bag. When reviewing a patient, IVN prescribers should take a brief look at any bag currently running to see if there may be an obvious problem.

If fitted, checking the bag and giving set for leaks (Plate 7a) or other damage (Plate 7b) is important as the bag would need to be discarded. This kind of damage can also occur during delivery and so all ward staff should inspect bags and giving sets before and during use (see Chapter 16).

Supplementary/independent prescribing and bag release (UK)

With the introduction of supplementary and independent prescribing (see Chapter 14), there is the possibility that a pharmacist prescriber could be responsible for the final release of a bag he or she prescribed. Although ideally this situation would not arise, there are various views as to whether it should be allowed. Prescribing and release-checking are quite different tasks: one is a clinical assessment whereas the other is primarily a technical assessment (Box 15.3). Furthermore, during the various Technical Services processes (Figure 15.1), many other staff will have been involved, providing additional safety. It therefore seems reasonable providing that the local system permits it and the individual pharmacist is comfortable with the process.

Technical Services' workload

Technical Services are responsible for compounding a number of products (Box 15.4) and so the workload of the Technical Services unit will clearly influence the provision of the IVN service because either fewer staff or a higher demand for any of the other product types compounded locally will limit the service that can be provided. It should also be clear that the time a prescription is received in Technical Services will affect their ability to deal with that request the same day (Figure 15.1).

Box 15.4 Examples of products compounded by Technical Services

Aseptic compounding
Intravenous feeds
Parenteral cytotoxics
Parenteral antibiotic doses
Others, e.g. trial products

Other products
Extemporaneous products e.g. creams, suspensions
Emergency drug kits

Note: the workload depends on all products for all patient groups (adults, paediatrics and neonates)

There may be occasions when the Technical Services unit is working at capacity and reasonable judgements must be made to ensure clinically appropriate but practical prescribing (see Chapter 11). All prescribed IVN regimens must include adequate micronutrients and, if there is no other option, consideration will need to be given to buying in regimens with micronutrients already added.

It is important to maintain good relations between Technical Services and the nutrition team and this requires an understanding of each other's role. The nutrition team pharmacist can be of great help here, but all IVN prescribers should visit their local Technical Services, and Technical Services' operators should be given the opportunity to obtain some practical experience of the nutrition team ward rounds. This collaboration allows more experience and mutual help with writing policies, e.g. for dealing with requests for emergency IVN (see Chapter 16), which affect both parties. The nutrition team can offer clinical considerations, with Technical Services contributing practical advice and help to implement developments.

Technical Services are often funded by directorates for the service provided. This offers various benefits, e.g. reduced pressure on ward staff and a strong element of risk management. Contracts should limit additional work without adequate funding and so collaboration with the nutrition team to ensure proper funding when new local developments increase workload is important (see Chapter 14).

Standardising bags and reducing wastage

Although it is important to tailor prescriptions for individual patients, this practice incurs considerable costs and creates extra work for Technical Services. You should therefore try to make the majority of your prescribing as similar as possible since this simplifies Technical Services routines. It also allows some bags to be reused in other patients when, for some reason, they are not used as originally intended (see Chapter 16). Electrolyte and micronutrient content in particular should be as standardised as possible, with higher or lower levels only prescribed if likely to grant significant clinical benefit (see Chapters 8 and 10).

It is always important to consider whether wasting the already compounded IVN can be avoided by taking simple measures to permit its use in the original patient or whether, with or without additional measures, it can be used in a different patient who currently needs IVN. However, if necessary, the bag should be discarded rather than used in a patient for whom it is unsuitable: the loss of a day's nutrition support poses a minimal risk compared to the dangers of giving an inappropriate regimen. Suitable measures to increase flexibility of regimen use include:

- *Separate supplemention of electrolytes that a patient needs in unusually large amounts*: although not through the same line lumen unless specifically confirmed as stable (see Appendix 1).
- *Reducing or increasing the rate of infusion*: which reduces or increases all elements of the provided IVN.

Contracting and local component stocks

Technical Services, in conjunction with the nutrition team, plays a key role in the IVN contracting process as well as in the decisions regarding which IVN components to stock locally.

Intravenous nutrition contracting

Nearly all hospitals have a contract with a specific manufacturer of IVN components, since contract prices always offer savings over list price. The components included in the contract should not be limited to precompounded and sterilised triple-chamber bags but should also include other bulk and more specialised components, along with the empty IVN bags that are needed for specially designed regimens. The contract price usually depends on the type and quantity of products that are used over a 12-month period.

It is usually necessary for manufacturers of IVN products to tender for IVN contracts. Tender specifications are produced by the hospital and must be specific to the proposed use and range of products needed. The contract should not prevent you from buying products from other suppliers if there is a clinical need but you will be obliged to place the majority of your orders with your main contractor. Purchase of products 'off-contract' will almost invariably be more expensive.

Companies will respond to invitations to tender with expressions of interest which are later followed by more detailed bids. Deciding on the company to be awarded the contract is never a decision to be made in isolation. Various staff need to be involved, including representatives from the nutrition team, members of Technical Services and pharmacy logistics, and hospital purchasing managers. The final decision is usually based on factors including:

- *Clinical value of products*: the reasons behind any clinically based decisions to favour one company's products over another must be clearly defined and justified and particular products must be specified by type, not brand. Remember to specify details in your contract specifications such as the ratios required for glucose to lipid energy. However, you have to be reasonable and should include a desirable range rather than, for example, the precise ratio of a particular supplier.

- *Range of products offered by a single supplier within the contract*: the more products that a company can supply, the fewer you will need to source off-contract at higher price. The ability to supply some products may be considered essential, e.g. empty IVN bags.

- *Technical merit of products offered*: there may be specific reasons why Technical Services needs particular products for use in the formulation of special regimens (see Chapter 11), e.g. a highly con-centrated nitrogen source for compounding low-volume regimens from basic components.

- *Support from the company*: a contracted company must be able to offer prompt support and stability advice and this may include support for commercial compounding software.

- *Logistics*: contracted companies must show that they will meet deadlines for orders and can obtain products swiftly when necessary.

- *Duration of contract*: changing contracts between suppliers involves significant work. An option to renew the contract without retendering may be included.
- *Added-value items*: offers of support for training or books are useful but may result in a higher price for the contract and can therefore be inappropriate.
- *The marketplace*: awarding a contract to a more expensive supplier in order to maintain competition in the marketplace is hard to justify but may prove useful in the longer term in order to avoid a monopoly.
- *Cost*: eventually cost is likely to be the deciding factor.

It may be beneficial to join forces locally or even nationally to achieve greater contract values and hence more competitive prices. All members of such a confederation must agree to the same contract terms. You will need to have documented evidence of agreement by all to the contract allocation along with a clear list of reasons why the contract was awarded to a particular supplier. Awarding the contract to multiple suppliers can occur but is likely to be complicated.

Local component stocks

Deliveries into your Technical Services unit need to be managed but there will usually be a departmental section that specialises in ensuring appropriate deliveries in response to requests for products. However, your local unit will not be able to stock every product available due to limited storage capacity, initial financial outlay and the risk of excessive wastage of expired products. It may also take some time to order in special requests.

It is therefore important to keep a sufficient range of products in stock to cater for the patients that you are likely to come across. In making this decision you will need to consider various factors including:

- *IVN purchasing contract*: this will determine from which of the major IVN component suppliers you will need to purchase the majority of your products. Note that you may not be able to obtain all your required products from this supplier, either because they do not supply them or because of a temporary lack of available stock for distribution.
- *Bulk macronutrients*: an appropriate range to allow required bags to be compounded when necessary (see Chapter 11).

- *Electrolyte salts for additions to IVN bags*: you will need to be able to prescribe additional electrolytes if required. Consider whether you need to stock more than one salt form (see Appendices 1 and 2).
- *Micronutrients*: you will require a complete range, including water-soluble and lipid-soluble vitamins and trace elements. Consider whether a specialist trace element preparation such as one without iron is to be used during the initial stages of IVN feeding (see Chapter 9) and your need for other specialist additions, such as Pabrinex, vitamin B_{12}, folic acid, copper sulphate, zinc sulphate and ascorbic acid (see also Appendix 3).
- *Precompounded triple-chamber bags*: for your usual patient range and numbers (see Chapter 11).

Technical Services licensing (UK)

All Technical Services units are strictly controlled by appropriate standards intended to protect the patients who will receive the compounded products. There are, however, three main types of licence status under which a unit may operate to aseptically compound products:

1. *Section 10 exemption (unlicensed)* can operate provided they comply with five conditions (Box 15.5).
2. *Specials licence* can compound batches without a prescription, can supply or sell to external customers (e.g. another hospital) and can assign any expiry to a product providing it can be justified. Specials units may also compound some products under section 10 exemption.
3. *Manufacturers' licence* is required for any product with a Marketing Authorisation (MA), formerly a Product Licence (PL).

Box 15.5 Technical Services section 10 exemption requirements[2]

1 Compounding is by or under the supervision of a pharmacist who takes full responsibility for the quality of the final product
2 Only licensed sterile medicinal starting materials or medicinal materials manufactured sterile in licensed facilities are used as ingredients
3 Only closed systems are used
4 Maximum expiry of 7 days (if justified)
5 Follow recommended guidance[3]

The Medicines and Healthcare products Regulatory Agency (MHRA), formerly known as the Medicines Control Agency (MCA), is the licensing authority in the UK.

IVN prescribers should at least be aware of the licence status of their local Technical Services unit, particularly because of the possibility of a 7-day limit on expiry of compounded products. This has implications for the timely reuse of unused bags where possible (see above). Home IVN regimens are usually compounded by a unit with a specials licence to allow a longer expiry when it can be justified.

References

1.   News. Two children die after receiving infected TPN solutions. *Pharm J* 1994; 252: 596.
2.   Beaney A, ed. *Quality Assurance of Aseptic Preparation Services*, 4th edn. London: Pharmaceutical Press, 2006: 1.
3.   Beaney A, ed. *Quality Assurance of Aseptic Preparation Services*, 4th edn. London: Pharmaceutical Press, 2006.

16

On the ward

Introduction

Although many checks have occurred by the time an intravenous nutrition (IVN) bag arrives on the ward, care is still needed if it is to be used safely and appropriately. Considerations include:

- Timing of planned IVN administration
- Starting and stopping IVN bags
- Managing intravenous access
- Special circumstances

Timing of intravenous nutrition administration

It is useful to have a consistent time for starting or swapping IVN bags to be sure of:

- *Availability of support*: in case of any queries and to ensure that the most appropriate skill mix of staff is on the ward at the time of administration. There should be enough staff to allow the time to use careful aseptic techniques.
- *Compounding and delivery of bags*: the IVN set-up time should take into account Technical Services workflow and should suit all concerned. If a bag runs out at an unusual time, the prescribing nutrition team or Technical Services may not be able to arrange for a replacement to be delivered when it is needed (see below).
- *Patient comfort*: patients do not want to be woken in the middle of the night to have a new bag of IVN started. Bags that run over less than 24 hours with a planned break should begin at a time that allows the break to be during the day.

A suggested workflow is shown in Figure 16.1, although the timings will need to be varied to suit local circumstances.

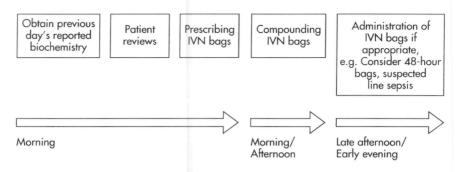

Figure 16.1 Simplified intravenous nutrition bag workflow.

With an appropriately agreed workflow (Figure 16.1), a new bag will usually be available when the previous one runs out. However, this may not always work in practice and if a new bag is likely to arrive late you can:

- Slow the rate of the current IVN infusion or
- Take the current bag down as soon as it is finished and flush the catheter lumen.

In either case, additional fluid and electrolytes may be required while waiting for the new bag to commence. If there is a delay in starting, it is often appropriate to disconnect the delayed bag before its completion, in order to recover the planned timing for changes with subsequent bags.

If, due to unforeseen circumstances, no bag is going to be available on a weekday, your only option is to give intravenous fluid and electrolyte provision as necessary to maintain the patient until the following day. At a weekend, if more than one bag has been prepared in advance, it may be possible to run a bag over 48 hours, although it is often simpler to miss a day of IVN. Patients prescribed IVN as an intermittent infusion (i.e. over less than 24 hours) should normally wait for the new bag to arrive whilst receiving fluids and electrolytes if necessary.

Starting an intravenous nutrition bag

Once an IVN bag has been delivered to the ward it should either be prepared for immediate use or the 'cold chain' (see Appendix 1) should be maintained.

Although the IVN will have been prescribed by a specialist, it is important that ward staff only give it if it is still needed and it is safe to do so. The most common reasons for concern would be:

- *Suspected intravenous catheter sepsis*: especially with an unexplained pyrexia of $\geq$ 38°C, as the risks usually outweigh the benefits of IVN in this situation. (N.B. not all patients will be pyrexial with line sepsis; see Chapter 12.)
- *Unplanned significant surgical intervention*: surgery exerts metabolic stress[1] and so for all significant operations or procedures it seems sensible to discontinue IVN immediately before the procedure and not to recommence it for at least 24 hours afterwards[2].
- *Failed placement of appropriate intravenous access*: need to await the placement, and confirmation of correct tip position if appropriate (see Chapter 12).
- *Progress on oral or enteral nutritional intake*: there may be occasions when the patient progresses more rapidly than expected and no longer requires the prescribed IVN (particularly if it is prescribed to commence a day or more after the patient was seen).
- *Significant change in the patient's fluid or electrolyte requirements*: changes in fluid and electrolyte needs can be sudden and pose a considerable risk to the patient, e.g. acute fluid overload or the development of acute renal failure with electrolyte retention.

If the use of prescribed IVN is delayed, remember to consider whether it should be commenced at a later stage.

Assuming it is appropriate to continue with the IVN as originally planned, the ward staff need to:

- *Check the bag integrity*: if there are any leaks, the microbiological risk is too great and the bag should not be used. Check the giving set for leaks or other damage (Plates 7a and 7b).
- *Check the bag fluid*: do not use if there are any signs of problems, e.g. precipitation (Plate 8).
- *Check the prescription against the bag label*: labelling errors are relatively common and so there should always be a check for discrepancies.

The purpose of the ward staff expressing concerns is not to undermine the prescriber but to take professional responsibility for administered medications. Most concerns are easily resolved and the prescriber will be grateful to learn of any problems. Clinical queries need to be raised with the nutrition team, a clinician responsible for the patient or, if necessary, the emergency duty pharmacist. Queries about the bag label should be raised with Technical Services (see Chapter 15) or the emergency duty pharmacist as they will have access to the compounding worksheets that show exactly what is in the bag.

If there are any doubts whether the patient should receive the feed and expert advice cannot be obtained, the only safe option is not to give it and to ensure that the patient is reviewed for intravenous fluids with or without electrolytes. The problem can then be discussed with the nutrition team on the next working day. In the case of queries on whether fluid and/or drugs can be given through the same line lumen as the IVN, the answer is no. If absolutely necessary, then the IVN will need to be discontinued to allow administration of other therapy. In this case, supplemental fluids with or without electrolytes as required may also need to be given (check stability of all products with each other before prescribing concurrent administration). Discuss with the nutrition team the next working day.

Missing a bag of IVN is not ideal but will not markedly affect nutritional status (but check blood glucose).

Warming the bag

Although compounded IVN should always be stored under refrigeration, it is inappropriate to administer a cold infusion and hence each bag should be warmed to room temperature before use. Warming should be achieved gradually by putting the bag on a work surface in the treatment room at ambient temperature for a period of 1–2 hours out of direct sunlight. Artificial heat, for example, placing the bag on a radiator or using a light source, should never be used since it poses a significant risk to bag stability.

Aseptic manipulation of the bag

The only acceptable aseptic manipulations of the bag on a ward are fitting a giving set to a bag *without* one already in place and connecting the bag to the patient's intravenous line for administration. It is critically important that:

- No additions are made to the bag because they may compromise the physical, chemical or microbiological stability (if the clinical situation has changed and additional electrolytes are now needed, they should be supplemented separately).

- No attempt is made to remove air or bubbles from the giving set with a needle and syringe.
- The giving set fitted in Technical Services is not changed (if the correct volumetric pump for the fitted giving set is not available, one will need to be borrowed or the IVN not given).

See also Chapter 15.

Commencing administration

Once the bag has been checked against the prescription and it is clear that it is the correct regimen and is still required (see above), full aseptic technique must be used to connect it to the patient's catheter. This limits the risks of catheter-related sepsis (see Chapter 12). A programmable volumetric pump with an in-line air alarm must be used to ensure accurate delivery of the required infusion rate and once the infusion is started, all appropriate documentation must be completed, e.g. signing of the prescription and entries on the fluid balance chart.

Sometimes patients on home IVN will require hospital admission, e.g. for intravenous catheter sepsis (see Chapter 12). If they are currently competent to do so (as assessed by the nutrition team) and depending on local policy, they may be able to connect and disconnect their own IVN, although they may be too ill to do so safely. Careful assessment and documentation are required.

'Emergency' intravenous nutrition

Nutrition is important but it should never be an emergency if proper planning is in place. Experience, however, shows that requests for emergency IVN are not uncommon.

Patients referred for emergency IVN are invariably very sick and are therefore at particular risk from inappropriate intravenous feeding. It is very unlikely that Technical Services (see Chapter 15) has the funding to permit individualised compounding of IVN bags out of normal working hours and this means that it is always the safest option to wait a day or two for IVN rather than commencing some sort of standard regimen without a formal nutritional assessment. Even worse is the use of a bag which lacks essential electrolytes and micronutrients (see Chapters 8 and 9). We therefore recommend that the emergency use of IVN should be avoided at any time, although a case can be made in very exceptional circumstances if the following day is not a normal

---

Box 16.1 Requirements for the use of emergency intravenous nutrition (IVN) (not recommended)

Ensure appropriate use
- Specific nutritional assessment (see Chapter 4)
- No specific contraindications, e.g. possible uncontrolled intravenous catheter sepsis (see Chapter 12)

Limit the risks of refeeding complications
- Adequate electrolytes in the IVN bag used
- Adequate micronutrients in the IVN bag used
- Slow introduction of IVN (i.e. very cautious rate)

Monitor for and correct any refeeding complications
- Patient is on a high-care or intensive care ward or can be transferred to such a ward before feeding

---

working day and there will be considerable delay before any nutrition can be provided.

Perception of 'exceptional circumstances' varies with who you ask, but if the patient is genuinely in need of emergency IVN, he or she must be sick enough to require consideration of the factors shown in Box 16.1.

Since all additions to an IVN bag should only be made in Technical Services (see Chapter 15), the only likely way that you can safely provide for emergency IVN is to keep bags with standard amounts of electrolytes and micronutrients already added, with access to them controlled by the emergency duty pharmacist. The content of these emergency regimens should be standardised (Box 16.2) and never kept as ward stock.

There should be no need to increase the rate of any emergency bag started outside normal working hours beyond quarter-rate or half-rate at most before a formal nutrition team assessment can be obtained on the next full working day. The aim should therefore be to use a single bag per patient, even if this means delaying the start by 24 hours in order that the regimen runs on into normal working hours. This will also limit the number of precompounded emergency bags that are kept at any one time. Occasionally, a long holiday weekend may justify more than one bag at half-rate or quarter-rate, hence the need for second bags to be available for 'emergency' patients.

Stopping intravenous nutrition

IVN is usually stopped when it is no longer needed and the patient can receive and tolerate adequate oral or enteral tube feeding. Once the

---

Box 16.2 Example of a precompounded 'emergency' intravenous nutrition bag

Nitrogen and energy
< 8 g nitrogen
< 1600 kcal (including nitrogen energy)

Electrolytes
Sodium: minimum practical content
Potassium: 120 mmol
Magnesium: 10 mmol
Calcium: 10 mmol
Phosphate: 35 mmol

Micronutrients
Water-soluble vitamins (double maintenance)
Lipid-soluble vitamins (double maintenance)
Trace elements (depending on product; see Chapter 9)

Rate of administration
Maximum half-rate or quarter-rate (see Chapter 7) for high-risk patients

Notes
All additions are subject to stability; make as close as possible.
Quarter-rate is likely to require additional separate potassium infusions.
Take care in patients with particular electrolyte requirements, e.g. renal failure.

---

patient begins to receive nutrition via the oral or enteral tube route then it is important to avoid overfeeding yet not discontinue IVN before another route is properly established. Prematurely stopping IVN may mean further nutritional depletion and risks of re-establishing IVN because the patient may not progress as hoped. If the central line has been routinely removed then a new one may be required. This is not without risks (see Chapter 12). Additionally there is likely to be a further workload resulting from the need to re-assess the patient for IVN.

In order to limit the potential for stopping IVN too early and to monitor for rebound hypoglycaemia, the IVN should usually be reduced to half-rate (see Chapter 7) before finally stopping. There may be occasions when this is not possible, such as when it is necessary to stop IVN in response to a suspected line sepsis, and in these cases careful monitoring of blood glucose is necessary.

When deciding whether to half-rate the IVN you will need to consider the nutritional value of any other intake. Tolerating water, jelly, icecream and usually also hospital soup by mouth is a good indication of progress but they do not provide complete nutrition. Once patients are able to take free fluids by mouth they should be prescribed oral sip supplements (lipid-free supplements if allowed clear free fluids). These can be very sweet and so are often diluted with milk (if they contain lipid) or water (if they are juice-based) to improve palatability. If oral intake is not possible or the patient lacks the volition for oral intake then enteral tube feeding should be considered.

Once the patient is tolerating 500 mL of nutritious fluids per day the IVN can be reduced to half-rate (see Chapter 7). Always ask patients if they are taking their sip supplements if these are prescribed and do not make an assumption that because they are offered them, they have successfully consumed all that have been prescribed. Oral or enteral tube feeding should be encouraged as permitted by the ward clinician to ensure that an adequate nutritional intake is tolerated before the IVN is finally stopped. This is likely to be half meals or the equivalent in oral sip supplements or enteral tube feed.

When you prescribe half-rate for a patient progressing off IVN you would not normally double up on electrolytes (see Chapter 11) because the other nutritious intake they receive should also contain electrolytes.

Unplanned stops in intravenous nutrition

There are some circumstances when, even though IVN is still needed, it has to be discontinued. This decision should be made by the nutrition team, a clinician or a qualified nurse. The most common reasons for unplanned stopping are:

- *Suspected intravenous catheter sepsis*: see Chapter 12.
- *Failed intravenous access*: e.g. the line has become blocked, fallen out or been pulled out.
- *Peripheral vein thrombophlebitis*: requiring midline removal (see Chapter 12).
- *Significant intervention*: as described in Chapter 3, surgery exerts metabolic stress, hence discontinuation of IVN before the operation and for 24 hours afterwards seems sensible.
- *Intravenous access required for other therapy*: it is not usually possible to run other fluids or drugs through the same lumen as IVN. If another therapy is more important in the short term, IVN may need to be discontinued (and the line flushed) to allow this to occur. Review by the nutrition team should take place on the next working day. IVN must never be reconnected once it has been disconnected due to the microbiological risks. Additional intravenous

fluids with or without electrolytes may be required until a new bag is available.

- *Significant change in the patient's fluid balance or electrolytes*: e.g. acute fluid overload or acute renal failure and changed electrolyte needs.

In any case where IVN is discontinued for any length of time, blood glucose should be monitored for rebound hypoglycaemia and any drugs to control blood glucose, especially insulin, will need urgent review.

Recommencing intravenous nutrition after an unplanned break

If, due to the problems mentioned above, a patient has their established, full-rate IVN interrupted, recommencement may sometimes require a step back to more modest levels of provision. This is probably unnecessary if the break in therapy is for less than 4 days and the patient had already received IVN at full-rate for several days before the break occurred and was clinically stable on a regimen. If, however, the gap is longer than 4 days, the IVN was never established at full-rate, or the patient was clinically unstable on the regimen given, recommencement at half-rate or even quarter-rate (see Chapter 7) may be needed, accounting for the same factors discussed in Chapters 7–11.

References

1.   Lobo D, Bostock K, Neal K *et al.* Effect of salt and water balance on recovery of gastrointestinal function after elective colonic resection: a randomised controlled trial. *Lancet* 2002; 359: 1812–1818.
2.   Buchman A. *Handbook of Nutritional Support.* Pennsylvania: Williams and Wilkins, 1997: 17–18.

Final note

Decisions on whether intravenous nutrition (IVN) is indicated, what to give and how to minimise risks and costs are as complex or more complex than prescribing in any other field. This book has aimed to cover all aspects, from the initial referral for IVN, through patient assessment and decisions on fluid, macronutrients and micronutrients, to watching for complications and organising your service. We have emphasised caution early on, suggesting that it is probably safer to provide only modest amounts of protein, fat and carbohydrate to a patient who has just entered the unstable 'metabolic chaos' of severe illness or injury. We have also suggested that generous amounts of electrolytes and micronutrients should be given at that time to meet the potentially abnormal needs and to correct any previous deficits. We recognise that there is little hard evidence for these suggestions, but in the absence of further research we believe that they have inherent logic.

This book concentrates on prescribing and makes no attempt to cover in depth the many other difficult issues, such as the complex nursing procedures, which are needed to minimise risks from catheter-related sepsis. We have, however, made some suggestions as to how we see nutrition teams working, stressing that in our opinion they should not make decisions from an office but should be out on the wards, visible, approachable and seeing the patients. Although beyond doubt, they should be multidisciplinary, that should not mean that roles are not shared. Indeed, this book was written with all members of multidisciplinary nutrition support teams in mind. Although it focuses on the processes of prescribing, it can hopefully contribute to each discipline's expertise and, even more importantly, help members of each discipline to understand the other's roles.

Peter Austin
Mike Stroud
December 2006

Appendix 1

Stability

Introduction

All prescribers of intravenous nutrition (IVN) must ensure the appropriate stability of any regimen they prescribe for a patient. Physical and chemical stability directly affect decisions the prescriber makes and appropriate microbiological stability is also essential. This is controlled using 'clean rooms'.

Once an IVN regimen has been compounded, a 'cold chain' must be maintained to ensure product quality when it is administered to the patient. Although maintaining the cold chain is typically within the remit of pharmacy for inpatients, all IVN prescribers should understand the requirement for a cold chain. This will allow them to make decisions on the reuse of in-hospital bags and to give informed advice to patients on home IVN. It will also permit informed interaction with commercial IVN suppliers.

Physical stability

Physical stability is concerned with ensuring no insoluble material forms (e.g. precipitate) and that the lipid component does not break down into free oil. Either of these is likely to result in blocking of the patient's vasculature following infusion and thus create a risk for thrombosis and pulmonary embolus.

Precipitation

Precipitates can form from an interaction between prescribed components such as electrolyte–electrolyte or electrolyte–trace element interactions. The potential for a precipitate to form is affected by a number of factors, including time, temperature, pH, salt type and concentration. The classical example of precipitation in IVN regimens is that arising from the addition of an excess of calcium and phosphate. It is possible

---

Box A1.1 Examples of some electrolyte salts

Inorganic salts
Sodium chloride
Disodium hydrogen phosphate
Potassium chloride
Potassium dihydrogen phosphate
Dipotassium hydrogen phosphate
Calcium chloride
Magnesium sulphate

Organic salts
Sodium acetate
Sodium glycerophosphate
Potassium acetate
Calcium gluconate

---

to include calcium and phosphate within an IVN regimen because the presence of all the other components allows them some space, but if the concentration is too high they will certainly precipitate. The stability risk of calcium phosphate precipitation is improved by amino acids, which decrease pH[1].

In view of the above, care must be taken to ensure adequate mixing of the bag after each addition and calcium or magnesium must never be added to the bag immediately before or after phosphate. Plate 8 shows the result of the sequential addition of calcium and phosphate to an IVN bag. If the bag had contained lipid, this may not have been detected, so it is important to have quality assurance systems in place to prevent this (see Chapter 15).

Organic salts (see Appendix 2) dissociate less in solution than inorganic salts and therefore greater quantities of electrolytes can often be added to IVN bags by using organic salts. Organic salts may also be used on some occasions to restrict electrolyte provision compared to an inorganic salt. For example, using sodium acetate does not provide chloride as well as sodium, in contrast to sodium chloride. Organic salts are typically more expensive than inorganic salts. Some examples of electrolyte salts are shown in Box A1.1.

The use of in-line filtration during IVN infusion may reduce the risk from precipitation but cannot replace accurate formulation and compounding.

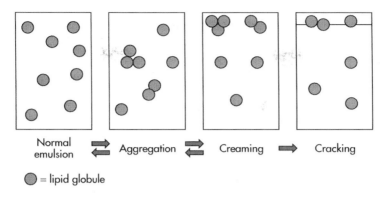

Figure A1.1 Lipid instability leading to cracking in intravenous feeds.

Lipid stability

Ordinarily lipid and water do not mix to form a continuous emulsion. However, the addition of a third component, an emulsifying agent, allows dispersion to occur. Commercially available IVN lipids contain an emulsifying agent as part of their formulation. As a consequence, excessive dilution of lipid in an IVN regimen will also dilute the available emulsifying agent to the point at which the quantity of emulsifying agent becomes insufficient to maintain the continuous phase and the lipid separates out.

Lipid may also separate out following the addition of large quantities of cationic electrolytes. This is because of disruption to the largely negative charge on the lipid globules, which allows the globules to come together. They then rise to the surface and form a 'cream', since the lipid is lighter than the aqueous phase. The lipid globules can sometimes be redispersed by shaking but if they become continuous, the lipid is said to have cracked and the change is irreversible (Figure A1.1). Reversible creaming is undesirable and cracking is dangerous, as the infusion of free oil can cause an embolism.

Chemical stability

Chemical stability is concerned with ensuring that the bioavailability of components within the IVN regimen is maintained. This can be difficult to measure and control. Chemical stability is important for, although the degradation products may not be harmful, the breakdown of components may mean that the patient does not receive the prescribed quantity. This explains why it is difficult to prescribe IVN regimens with

---

Box A1.2 Influences on chemical stability of intravenous nutrition regimens

Light
Light speeds up reactions, e.g. ultraviolet photodegradation of vitamin A if the patient is near a window

Temperature
Higher temperatures speed up reaction rates (usually including microbiological growth)

Oxygen
Oxygen causes oxidation reactions to occur, e.g. begins the breakdown of ascorbic acid. Do not allow too much air into the bag during compounding as this will form an oxygen reservoir. For bags with added micronutrients that require a longer expiry date, extra ascorbic acid may be added to act as an oxygen scavenger and to ensure sufficient is available at the time of use

Trace elements
Trace elements can act as catalysts

Container
Polyvinyl chloride (PVC) is unsuitable due to leaching of plasticisers. Ethylene vinyl acetate (EVA) is a poor oxygen barrier so ideally multilayer oxygen-impermeable bags should be used

---

added micronutrients and expect them to remain stable for prolonged periods after they are compounded.

Various factors, including light and heat, can influence chemical stability (Box A1.2) and as a result all compounded regimens should be protected from light and kept in a refrigerator until required (unless terminally sterilised and stable). Bags stored in a refrigerator should be gently warmed to room temperature before use (see Chapter 16).

Some centres only light-protect lipid-free regimens, relying on the lipid in the bag to protect the other components. The problem with this approach is that the lipid itself can be attacked by the light, resulting in lipid peroxidation and the generation of free radicals. There is therefore an argument for protecting all IVN regimens from light, whether they contain lipid or not.

Assessing the stability of intravenous nutrition regimens

In view of the many potential problems discussed above, you must always ensure the stability of an IVN regimen that you prescribe. As well as standard prescribing you should therefore know how to approach questions of including drugs within IVN bags and you should understand when drugs and/or fluid can be administered concurrently through the same lumen as the IVN. Although both practices should generally be avoided, there may be circumstances where they must be considered and the safety of permitting such practices will depend, at least in part, on the specific IVN regimen prescribed.

Standard prescribing

Commercial manufacturers of IVN components are able to supply standard stability tables for their range of products. These tables will show the maximum quantity of each common addition to their range of standard triple-chamber bags (see Chapter 11) and can also provide guidance on regimens created to meet individual patients' needs. Always ensure that you are clear whether the stability data relate to the total bag quantity or the concentration per litre.

Occasionally you will need to prescribe a regimen that is not covered by the standard stability tables, in which case you will need to

---

Box A1.3 Basic guidelines on intravenous nutrition (IVN) stability applicable in many circumstancest

Magnesium can be increased at the expense of calcium but not beyond the total calcium and magnesium permitted. This is not the case the other way round, e.g. limits of 5 mmol (total) of each means 8 mmol magnesium and up to 2 mmol calcium may be possible but calcium is very likely to be restricted to 5 mmol regardless of the quantity of any magnesium present

Different manufacturers may not take the same view regarding the phosphate contribution from the lipid. It is always simplest to assume that it is included in the total phosphate in the regimen, but this must be clear during discussions

Avoid mixing macronutrient products between companies

Lipids of the same general type (e.g. 100% long-chain triglyceride-based (see Chapter 7) of the same concentration) are often interchangeable for stability purposes

It is likely that the addition of water-soluble vitamins, such as folic acid injection, to IVN bags will be stable

Note: These guidelines do not apply in all circumstances and you must always obtain confirmation of stability from the manufacturer before prescribing

contact the manufacturer directly to discuss your requirements. However, it is often the case that observing a few guidelines can save you time (Box A1.3), even although you will still need to obtain written confirmation of stability (e.g. a headed fax) before prescribing any IVN regimen which is not included in standard tables.

Incorporating drugs within intravenous nutrition regimens

Adding a drug to an IVN regimen may be helpful in order to limit the fluid and/or electrolyte load the patient receives. It can also limit the number of aseptic manipulations needed in the clinical environment and solve problems related to lack of intravenous access. Occasionally, the addition may be intended as an integral part of the regimen, e.g. to limit peripheral vein thrombophlebitis (see Chapter 12), although this is not recommended. Since there are several potential problems related to adding a drug to an IVN bag (Box A1.4), it should only be done if there is both a clear benefit and evidence of appropriate stability.

The inclusion of insulin within IVN regimens to promote anabolism has been considered, but there are many drawbacks, including metabolic disturbances[2]. We do not recommend the administration of insulin with this intention.

Box A1.4 Potential problems of adding drugs to intravenous nutrition (IVN) regimens

---

Stability
Of the IVN, e.g. precipitation with aciclovir or 'cracking' with heparin
Of the added drug – remaining active quantity may be limited

Infusion duration
Rate of administration (drug versus IVN) – which takes priority? e.g. insulin with high blood glucose – do you increase the rate of IVN, which will give a higher glucose load as well as more insulin?

Drug availability
For example, insulin can adsorb on to the plastics in the bag and giving set variably, limiting availability to the patient for the same IVN prescription

The added drug may need to be stopped following compounding of several IVN bags incorporating it

Note: adding more than one drug to an IVN bag complicates this even more – extreme caution and highly specialist advice are required

---

Before any drug is added to an IVN bag, evidence of stability from the manufacturer or from another source, such as 'Trissel'[3], is required. 'Trissel' requires very careful interpretation since it may not include the regimen that you require. Nevertheless, it can indicate whether a particular addition is obviously inappropriate or whether further investigations are warranted. Always seek specialist advice before prescribing any drug to be added to an IVN regimen.

Concurrently administering drugs and/or fluid through the intravenous nutrition lumen

Administration of any drug and/or fluid through the same lumen as IVN must be avoided if possible, although some circumstances may mean that this option has to be considered. If the proposed infusate will come into physical contact with the IVN (see Figure 12.2 in Chapter 12), you will need supporting stability data before concurrent administration.

Concurrent administration of fluids and/or electrolytes requires you to know the maximum permitted fluid and relevant electrolyte additions to the prescribed IVN regimen (see above). You then work out the maximum fluid rate and electrolyte content of the separate infusion by assuming that the separate infusion has been added to the IVN regimen during compounding.

The concurrent infusion of drugs is more complex as it depends on additional factors, e.g. the concentration of the drug infusate. Supporting data may be available from the manufacturer, the literature or from a source such as 'Trissel'[3]. Always be very careful how any information is interpreted.

Microbiological stability

The infusion of micro-organisms directly into a patient's vein bypasses natural defences and can make patients very sick. It can even be fatal[4]. IVN is an ideal growth medium for many micro-organisms and even a single introduced contaminant can rapidly multiply into a very significant infection. This means that it is critically important to ensure this does not happen, particularly as compounded IVN bags may be stored before administration to a patient and then infused over a long period at ambient temperature (sometimes up to 48 hours).

Aseptic technique can be defined as the 'manipulation of (sterile) starting materials in such a way so as to minimise the risk of contamination of the final product'. Aseptic technique can be good or poor and

---

Box A1.5 Techniques used to improve microbiological stability

Use of terminally sterilised triple-chamber bags
The fewer aseptic manipulations the better, but not at the expense of
appropriate formulation

*Intravenous nutrition (IVN) compounded within dedicated pharmacy clean
rooms (see text and Chapter 15)*
The less environmental contamination, the lower the risk of incorporating
micro-organisms in the final product by chance (see text)

Strict aseptic technique to compound all IVN bags
Only dedicated and validated operators should be permitted to compound
IVN regimens for patients (see Chapter 15)

An appropriate cold chain is maintained (see text)
Once aseptically compounded, or additions have been made, all IVN bags
must be kept under refrigeration until required once additions have been
made

---

can be carried out in a variety of settings. In all cases, however, contamination of the prepared product remains possible as there is always
an element of chance.

Microbiological stability is concerned with preventing the presence
(and growth) of bacteria and fungi along with the toxins produced by
micro-organisms. Viruses are obligate intracellular parasites and are
therefore not considered a risk to compounded IVN bags. Box A1.5
shows various techniques that can be used to improve the microbiological stability of compounded IVN bags.

Clean-room design

A clean room is a room designed to minimise the level of viable, non-
viable and particulate contamination present. Within this room is a
cabinet in which prescribed IVN regimens are compounded in the
'critical zone' (Plate 5). This minimises the risk that any contamination
that is present in the room is incorporated into the bag during the
compounding process (Figure A1.2).

All clean rooms have numerous features to minimise the amount
of contamination within the room. These features include:

- *Smooth, easily cleanable surfaces*: to minimise the risk of microbiological contamination 'hiding' in difficult-to-access areas that

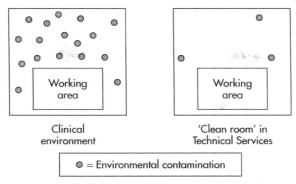

A higher level of background contamination increases the risk
of it being incorporated into the final product by chance

Figure A1.2 Minimising contamination of products prepared in Technical Services
compared to a clinical environment by limiting background contamination.

can then be transferred to the critical zone (e.g. on a floating
particle).

- *Air intake*: the dedicated air-handling plant minimises the risk of
  contaminated air entering the room. This is achieved by passing
  the air through a series of filters, beginning with a very large pore
  size and finishing with a high-efficiency particulate air (HEPA) filter
  of 0.2 micron pore size immediately.
- *Positive pressure*: generated by the air intake (above) means that
  even when a door is opened, the only air that can enter the room
  is that originating from the air-handling plant. This limits contamination entering the room.
- *Specific room airflow pattern*: to aim to 'wash away' any contamination in difficult-to-clean areas.
- *Cabinet HEPA filters*: the air intake to the cabinets passes through
  a further HEPA filter to keep the air as free from contamination as
  possible.
- *Specific cabinet airflow pattern*: depends on the type of cabinet
  used, but generally forces air away from the critical zone. This
  airflow pattern dictates the correct aseptic technique to be used in
  a particular cabinet to maximise clean air flowing over the highest-
  risk areas (e.g. injection ports). The cabinet will also have either a
  physical barrier or 'air curtain' to prevent any air reaching the
  product that has not gone through the cabinet filter.

Use of clean rooms

Access to clean rooms is restricted in order to maintain the integrity of the system and avoid introducing contaminants into the environment.

All products are sprayed and/or wiped into the clean room and then again into the cabinet, e.g. with 70% alcohol to kill and/or remove any microbiological contamination. Clutter, e.g. packaging, packaging waste and especially other products, is always avoided to limit the risks of error, cross-contamination and microbiological transfer on particles.

All operators who work within a clean room are thoroughly trained and validated to use a consistent aseptic technique that minimises the risk to the product.

Operator assessment is typically carried out in the form of a broth test[5], which involves various aseptic manipulations of a growth medium to present a worst-case scenario (Plate 9). If there is any growth in prepared products or a poor technique, the operator fails the test. A dye may be used during some of the manipulations to show more easily poor technique, e.g. spills or sprays.

When working, operators must move carefully within the room to minimise disruption to airflow (see above) that might dislodge contaminants (Box 15.2). The aseptic technique that is adopted depends on the cabinet design, with the aim of giving maximum airflow in the critical zone, where the product is actually compounded. Additions are often double-checked before they are put into a bag (depending on local policy) and they must enter the bag in a suitable order, e.g. calcium and phosphate must be separated with adequate mixing between each addition to avoid precipitation (Plate 8). Given a choice, electrolytes are added before lipid so that any precipitation can be seen (see above).

The repeated movements of drawing up IVN additions are time-consuming and can put a strain on the operators, particularly if a poor aseptic technique is used. This can ultimately lead to repetitive strain injury. It is therefore important to ensure a comfortable working position and regular rest breaks from repetitive tasks. Clinically irrelevant electrolyte additions should be avoided. Automation of some processes may be possible but, although a great increase in speed may be obtained, it can be expensive, complex to validate and time-consuming to set up.

The operators are also trained in the appropriate monitoring, cleaning and use of the clean room. Monitoring for microbiological (as well as particulate) contamination is regularly required to ensure that standards are met and is an important aspect of patient safety. Regular

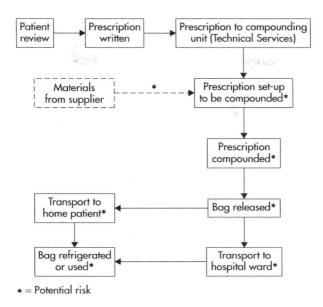

Figure A1.3 Risks to the cold chain of intravenous nutrition regimens.

cleaning limits the build-up of contamination and includes all surfaces, e.g. walls and ceilings, as well as the cabinets. All operators and approved visitors must wear special clean-room clothing (Plate 5) to minimise natural shedding of micro-organisms and particles. The clothing design will depend on the specifics of the local clean room.

Delivery and the cold chain

IVN bags and components are often temperature-sensitive (see above) and so compounded regimens must always be refrigerated when not in use. The only exception is immediately before administration (see Chapter 16). It is therefore essential to ensure appropriate continuation of the cold chain (Figure A1.3).

Once an IVN bag has been released for administration to the patient it must be transported to the patient's location before it can be used. The many risks to the cold chain shown in Figure A1.3 must be controlled in order to maintain the stability of compounded IVN regimens.

The cold chain in intravenous nutrition compounding

Potential problems can arise at any phase of product compounding and delivery to the patient:

- *During original compounding*: all reputable manufacturers of IVN components have systems in place to maintain an appropriate cold chain similar to those for locally compounded IVN bags (see below).
- *During IVN compounding*: all IVN compounding units must ensure that they have appropriate systems to keep to a minimum the time at ambient temperature of all components requiring refrigeration. Workflow must be planned and validated to minimise warming risks.
- *Delays in release of compounded bags*: a shortage of pharmacists with appropriate skills in Technical Services and IVN compounding can result in delays in checking compounded IVN bags. Leaving compounded bags at ambient temperature while awaiting release is not an acceptable practice and if delays are likely, the compounded bags should be stored in quarantine under refrigeration until release-checking is performed. The quarantine system must ensure that only appropriately released bags can leave the unit.
- *Difficulties in refrigerating compounded bags*: once a bag has been released, the possibility of further refrigeration before transport to the ward should be considered. This is particularly true if delays in transport are likely, or the use of large volumes of non-refrigerated components in the regimen has led to the production of bags which are already close to room temperature. However, arranging to cool large volumes of IVN is not easy and, although compounding IVN using refrigerated bulk components limits the problem, it can create another. Condensation on the outside of cold bags within compounding cabinets introduces moisture to the compounding facilities that then increases the risks of microbiological contamination.

The cold chain during on-site delivery and use

Maintaining the IVN cold chain after the bags leave Technical Services is equally important in maintaining stability of the regimens. A variety of factors need consideration to limit the warming threats during delivery within a hospital:

- *Type, size and quantity of IVN bags*: this will affect packaging arrangements, size of delivery vehicle or number of journeys and time to each destination if more than one.
- *Type, size and quantity of cool packs*: ability to chill will depend on the type, size and quantity of cool packs in relation to the number, size, arrangement and initial temperature of the IVN bags.
- *Packaging arrangements*: each arrangement of bags and cool packs will affect the ability of the cool packs to chill the IVN bags adequately.
- *Delivery distance*: consider whether any delays are likely and how long they might be. For more than one delivery destination, consider all individual destinations and the effects of unloading previous deliveries on the temperature control of the subsequent deliveries.
- *Weather and time of year*: particularly important for external deliveries but also relevant to deliveries across a site where the product is exposed to the weather.
- *What happens to the IVN when it arrives*: consider if there might be a delay in refrigeration and if so, how long this might be for. For example, for busy hospital wards you may need to look at appropriate education of ward and portering staff to refrigerate delivered bags or consider validation of the use of cool packs for internal deliveries.
- *When the IVN will arrive*: consider whether any queries can be easily resolved on arrival and whether the delivery should be confirmed to prevent inappropriate warming of bags or to allow a contingency plan to be actioned if necessary. Accurate and timely delivery is important to ensure that someone is available to receive the delivered bags, allowing the subsequent maintenance of the cold chain.

The cold chain during off-site delivery

For long-distance deliveries a validated specialist company is often a useful, but costly, option. They should, however, be able to supply a print-out of the product temperature during transport. For longer-distance deliveries in a van, consider that the sunshine warming the internal areas of the van is likely to be more relevant than the external ambient temperature.

References

1. Shulman R, Reed T, Pitre D, Laine L. Use of hydrochloric acid to clear obstructed central venous catheters. *J Parenteral Enteral Nutr* 1998; 12: 509–510.
2. Woolfson A. The use of insulin in intravenous nutrition. In: Karran S, Alberti K, eds. *Practical Nutritional Support*. London: Pitman Medical, 1980: 160–165.
3. Trissel L. *Handbook on Injectable Drugs*. Bethseda: American Society of Health-System Pharmacists, 2005.
4. Farwell, J. *Aseptic Dispensing for NHS Patients*. London: Department of Health, 1995.
5. Beaney A, ed. *Quality Assurance of Aseptic Preparation Services*, 4th edn. London: Pharmaceutical Press, 2006: 93–94.

Appendix 2

Salts and pharmaceutical calculations

Introduction

All intravenous nutrition (IVN) prescribers should understand the effects of using different salts within the regimens they prescribe, since this can directly affect stability and may influence decisions on which electrolytes to add.

Being able to perform calculations with the commonly used units of concentration and measurement is also important it enables you to convert between different units that are used, permitting the design of regimens from basic components.

Salts

A salt is the compound formed when the hydrogen of an acid is replaced, either entirely or partly, by a metal. A salt is made up of two or more ionic species (also called ions). Each ionic species is an atom or molecule with either an excess or deficit of electrons. It therefore has a charge. This charge will be negative (excess of electrons) or positive (deficit of electrons) and is described by the common oxidation (or valency) number of the atom or molecule (Table A2.1). A positive ion is called a cation and a negative ion is called an anion.

Table A2.1 Table of common oxidation numbers

Oxidation number	Examples
−3	Phosphate (PO_4)
−2	Sulphate (SO_4), oxygen (O)
−1	Chloride (Cl), bicarbonate (HCO_3)
+1	Sodium (Na), potassium (K), hydrogen (H)
+2	Magnesium (Mg), calcium (Ca), iron(II) (Fe(II))
+3	Iron(III) (Fe(III))

Dipotassium hydrogen phosphate

Potassium dihydrogen phosphate

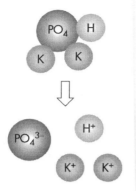

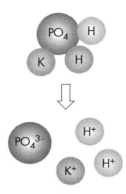

Prescribing 1 mmol phosphate adds
2 mmol potassium (and 1 mmol hydrogen)

Prescribing 1 mmol phosphate adds
1 mmol potassium (and 2 mmol hydrogen)

Figure A2.1 The examples of potassium phosphate show the importance of being clear which salts are stocked locally.

Some ionic species exist in different states that have different oxidation numbers, e.g. iron. It is usual practice to assume an oxidation number of 2 for these species unless specified otherwise but always check.

All common electrolyte additions to IVN regimens consist of a salt, e.g. sodium chloride or potassium phosphate. The addition of one electrolyte will therefore lead to the addition of other ions. You should be aware of the precise salts that are stocked locally (Figure A2.1).

The nature and quantity of additional electrolytes that you add to your IVN regimen will therefore depend on:

- *The components of the salt used*: the different electrolyte salts will dictate which other ions are added when prescribing a particular electrolyte addition.
- *The oxidation numbers of the ionic species in the salt used*: the ratio between the components will determine how much of each will be added per unit volume.

The required volume of a salt needed to give a specified quantity of a particular electrolyte will depend on the concentration of the salt preparation stocked.

In addition to influencing the electrolytes added to your bag, the type of salt you use can affect the stability of the IVN regimen depending whether it is organic or inorganic.

Organic salts are weak, meaning that there is relatively limited dissociation of the component ions in solution, whereas inorganic salts are strong, meaning that there is very high (if not complete) dissociation of their component ions when dissolved. Since it is dissociated free ions that react, organic salts are more stable than inorganic salts. However, they are usually more expensive and are therefore only used when necessary.

Standard IVN stability tables (see Appendix 1) usually assume that you use inorganic salts, but you should always check this before prescribing. If the table does assume the use of inorganic salts, the manufacturer may be able to offer stability for even greater electrolyte additions using organic salts.

There are many different electrolyte salts available to help control, at least to an extent, the nature and quantity of additional electrolytes you are forced to add. For example, in order to limit phosphate additions you could use sodium chloride rather than sodium glycerophosphate subject to stability (Table A2.2).

Adding phosphate usually adds at least one other electrolyte. For example, using Addiphos will add phosphate, sodium and potassium in the ratio 2 mmol phosphate to 1.5 mmol of each of sodium and potassium. This means that by adding Addiphos you must adjust the quantities of sodium and potassium in your regimen whether you want to or not. If this is not suitable then your options include:

• Add less Addiphos and therefore less sodium and potassium (accepting the lower phosphate provision)
• Use a different phosphate salt (but note that you will have to add either sodium or potassium and possibly more of it than with Addiphos)
• Add no phosphate to the IVN regimen (accepting the lower phosphate provision)

You may occasionally wish to restrict the chloride content of your IVN regimen, in which case you will need to consider the use of non-chloride salts.

Units of concentration and measurement

The basic units of concentration and measurement that you come across within IVN services are usually millimoles and percentages, although you may also see milliequivalents and grams, e.g. potassium prescribed as grams of potassium chloride in intravenous infusions. You therefore

Table A2.2 Examples of salts you may use when adding electrolytes to your intravenous nutrition regimen

Intended electrolyte addition	Examples of salt options	Option will provide (approximate mmol per mL)	Organic or inorganic salt*
Sodium	30% w/v sodium chloride	5.13 sodium 5.13 chloride	Inorganic
	30% w/v sodium acetate	2.2 sodium 2.2 acetate	Organic
	21.6% w/v sodium glycerrophosphate	2 sodium 1 phosphate	Organic
	Addiphos	(see below)	Inorganic
Potassium	15% w/v potassium chloride	2 potassium 2 chloride	Inorganic
	20% w/v potassium chloride	2.68 potassium 2.68 chloride	Inorganic
	49% w/v potassium acetate	5 potassium 5 acetate	Organic
	13.6% w/v potassium dihydrogen phosphate	1 potassium 1 phosphate	Inorganic
	17.42% w/v dipotassium hydrogen phosphate	2 potassium 1 phosphate	Inorganic
	Addiphos	(see below)	Inorganic
Magnesium	50% w/v magnesium sulphate	2 magnesium 2 sulphate	Inorganic
Calcium	14.7% w/v calcium chloride	1 calcium 2 chloride	Inorganic
	10% w/v calcium gluconate	0.22 calcium	Organic
Phosphate	Addiphos	2 phosphate 1.5 sodium 1.5 potassium	Inorganic
	13.6% w/v potassium dihydrogen phosphate	1 potassium 1 phosphate	Inorganic
	17.42% w/v dipotassium hydrogen phosphate	2 potassium 1 phosphate	Inorganic

* The difference between an organic and an inorganic salt is explained in the text.

need an understanding of each of these units in order to compare different products and to be able to formulate your own regimens (see Chapter 11).

Table A2.3 Common atomic masses used in Technical Services

Element	Element symbol	Approximate atomic mass*
Calcium	Ca	40.1
Carbon-12	C	12
Chloride	Cl	35.5
Copper	Cu	63.5
Hydrogen	H	1
Magnesium	Mg	24
Oxygen	O	16
Phosphorus	P	31
Potassium	K	39
Selenium	Se	79
Sodium	Na	23
Sulphur	S	32
Zinc	Zn	65

* Note that you may need to add up individual atomic masses depending on the formula with which you are working, e.g. phosphate is PO_4 (1 phosphorus plus 4 oxygens with a total molecular mass of 95) or dipotassium is K_2 (2 potassium atoms with a total mass of 78) but potassium is K (1 potassium with an atomic weight of 39).

Millimoles

One mole of any substance contains approximately 6.023×10^{23} atoms (Avogadro's number) and its weight is the same as the atomic mass of that substance expressed in grams on a scale where 1 mole of carbon-12 weighs 12 g.

Some common atomic masses used in Technical Services are shown in Table A2.3. These are useful for the example calculations below.

One millimole is one thousandth of a mole (Equation A2.1).

$$(1 \text{ millimole}) = (1 \text{ mole})/(1000) \tag{Eqn A2.1}$$

Percentages

Glucose, lipids and electrolytes are available in different concentrations, which may be expressed in percentage terms. A percentage concentration means:

- The number of grams per 100 g or
- The number of grams per 100 mL or
- The number of millilitres per 100 g or
- The number of millilitres per 100 mL

This means that, rather than simply referring to %, technically you should add w/w, w/v, v/w or v/v after it, where w refers to weight and v refers to volume.

However, when discussing nutritional regimens and requirements, you must also be aware that percentages of macronutrients often refer to the percentage of energy (in kilocalories or kilojoules) provided by that macronutrient in relation to the total energy provision.

Milliequivalents

Milliequivalents are the equivalent weight of combining atoms in a reaction and are dependent on the oxidation number of the relevant ion (see above), as shown in Equation A2.2[1].

(milliequivalents) = (mmol) $\times$ (oxidation number, ignoring charge)

(Eqn A2.2)

If the ion has an oxidation number of 1, then the number of milliequivalents will be equal to the number of millimoles.

Grams

A gram is a unit of mass that is simply converted to milligrams (Equation A2.3).

(1 gram) = (1000 milligrams) (Eqn A2.3)

Pharmaceutical calculations

Being able to use and convert between different units is a great advantage to the IVN prescriber.

The key concept with percentages is that a percentage means the number of grams or millilitres per 100 g or 100 mL of product. Understanding this will allow you to convert between different formulations.

Equation A2.4 is very useful for converting between moles and grams, but you will still need to consider the information above.

(moles) = (mass in grams)/(molecular weight) (Eqn A2.4)

Always be clear of the molecular formula with which you are working and whether it has any water of crystallisation, i.e. it contains water which adds to the total molecular weight. You can find out the molecular formula and whether there is any water of crystallisation in the *British*

Pharmacopoeia for products specified as 'BP' (they meet the *British Pharmacopoeia* standard)[2].

When working with a molecular formula containing two ionic species (above) that are in a ratio of 1:1 (their oxidation numbers are the same but of opposite charge; Table A2.1), using Equation A2.4 the number of moles will be the mass in grams divided by the total molecular weight. Otherwise you will need to work out how much of the molecule consists of the electrolyte you are interested in before using the molecular weight for that electrolyte alone in Equation A2.4. See the examples below and those in Appendix 4.

Example 1

You wish to convert 1000 mL intravenous infusion containing 0.2% w/v potassium chloride into mmol of potassium in 1000 mL.

1. 0.2% w/v potassium chloride is 0.2 g potassium chloride in 100 mL. In 1000 mL you have (0.2 g/100) × 1000 = 2 g potassium chloride.
2. Using Table A2.3 and Equation A2.4, 2 g potassium chloride is (2)/(39 + 35.5) = 0.0268 moles which is (0.0268) × (1000) = 26.8 or 27 mmol potassium in 1000 mL.

Note that the mmol of potassium and chloride are the same because the oxidation numbers of each are both 1 (Table A2.1). This calculation would be different if you were using calcium chloride, where the oxidation numbers of the salt components are different (see next example).

Example 2

You wish to convert 14.7% w/v calcium chloride into mmol per 10mL.

1. 14.7% w/v is equivalent to 14.7 g in 100 mL. Each calcium ion is associated with two chloride ions, as the formula is $CaCl_2$ using Table A2.1. Calcium chloride is also associated with 2 water molecules of crystallisation[3], making the formula $CaCl_2.2H_2O$. Both of these mean that you need to calculate the proportion of the total mmol attributable to calcium. You do this using the atomic weights from Table A2.3. So the total weight of calcium chloride is 40.1 + 35.5 + 35.5 + 1 + 1 + 1 + 1 + 16 + 16 = 147.1. Calcium represents (40.1/147.1) × 100 = 27.3% of the total. So (27.3/100) × 14.7 = 4.013 g calcium in 100 mL of calcium chloride.

2. Using Equation A2.4, 4.013 g calcium is (4.013)/(40.1) = 0.100 moles which is (0.100) × (1000) = 100 mmol in 100 mL. This is equivalent to (100)/(10) = 10 mmol calcium in 10 mL of 14.7% w/v calcium chloride.

Example 3
You wish to convert 1000 mL intravenous infusion containing 2 g potassium chloride into mmol of potassium in 1000 mL.

1. Using Equation A2.4, 2 g potassium chloride is (2)/(39 + 35.5) = 0.0268 moles which is (0.0268) × (1000) = 26.8 or 27 mmol potassium in 1000 mL.

Note that the mmol of potassium and chloride are the same because the oxidation numbers of each are both 1 (Table A2.1). This calculation would be different if you were using calcium chloride, where the oxidation numbers of the salt components are different (see previous example).

Example 4
You wish to convert 27 mmol potassium in 1000 mL into % w/v potassium chloride.

1. Using the chloride salt, 27 mmol potassium is the same as 27 mmol potassium chloride because the oxidation numbers of potassium and chloride are both 1 (Table A2.1) and there is no water of crystallisation. Rearranging Equation A2.4 and using Table A2.3, 27 mmol potassium chloride = (27) × (39 + 35.5) = 2012 mg or (2012)/(1000) = 2.012 g potassium chloride.
2. For % w/v you need the number of grams per 100 mL = (2.012)/(1000) × 100 = 0.201 or 0.2% w/v.

Example 5
You wish to convert 60 mmol of potassium in 1000 mL into grams of potassium chloride in 1000 mL.

1. Using the chloride salt, 60 mmol potassium is the same as 60 mmol potassium chloride because the oxidation numbers of both potassium and chloride are both 1 (Table A2.1). Rearranging Equation A2.4 and using Table A2.3, 60 mmol potassium chloride = (60) × (39 + 35.5) = 4470 mg or (4470)/(1000) = 4.47 or 4.5 g potassium chloride in 1000 mL.

Example 6

Consider whether 500 mL of 20% w/v lipid and 333 mL of 30% w/v lipid contain the same number of grams of lipid.

1. 500 mL of 20% w/v lipid would provide 20 g lipid per 100 mL. The concentration is 20 g/100 mL = 0.2 g/mL. In 500 mL we have 500 mL × 0.2 g/mL = 100 g lipid.
2. 333 mL of 30% w/v lipid would provide 30 g lipid per 100 mL. The concentration is 30 g/100 mL = 0.3 g/mL. In 333 mL we have 333 mL × 0.3 g/mL = 99.9 g lipid (round up to 100 g lipid).

Therefore 500 mL of 20% w/v lipid and 333 mL of 30% w/v lipid are equivalent in grams of lipid provision despite varying in both concentration and volume.

Example 7

You wish to convert 20 mmol potassium into milliequivalents.

1. The oxidation number of potassium is +1 (Table A2.1) so, using Equation A2.2, 20 mmol is (20) × (1) = 20 mEq.

Example 8

You wish to convert 10 mmol phosphate into milliequivalents.

1. The oxidation number of phosphate is –3 (Table A2.1) so, using Equation A2.2, 10 mmol is (10) × (3) = 30 mEq.

Example 9

You wish to convert 10 mEq of calcium into mmol.

1. The oxidation number of calcium is +2 (Table A2.1) so, rearranging Equation A2.2, 10 mEq is (10)/(2) = 5 mmol.

Example 10

You wish to know how many milliequivalents of each of potassium and phosphate there are in 10 mL of 17.42% w/v dipotassium hydrogen phosphate.

1. 17.42% dipotassium hydrogen phosphate has the formula K_2HPO_4 and has a total molecular weight of 174 (from Table A2.3). 17.42% dipotassium hydrogen phosphate is 17.42 g of dipotassium hydrogen phosphate in 100 mL. There are two potassium atoms with a molecular weight of (39 × 2) = 78. There

is therefore $((78)/(174)) \times (100) = 44.8\%$ of the 17.42 g in 100 mL as potassium which is $((44.8)/(100)) \times 17.42 = 7.80$ g potassium.

2. Using Equation A2.4, there are $(7.8)/(39) = 0.20$ moles of potassium in 100 mL. Note that it is not appropriate to double up the atomic weight of potassium here.

3. 0.20 moles potassium in 100 mL is $(0.20) \times (1000) = 200$ mmol potassium in 100 mL or $((200)/(100)) \times (10) = 20$ mmol potassium in 10 mL of 17.42% w/v dipotassium hydrogen phosphate.

4. Using Equation A2.2, this is $(20) \times (1) = 20$ mEq of potassium in 10 mL of 17.42% w/v dipotassium hydrogen phosphate.

5. There is 1 phosphate with a molecular weight of $((31) + (16 \times 4)) = 95$. There is therefore $((95)/(174)) \times (100) = 54.6\%$ of the 17.42 g in 100 mL as phosphate which is $((54.6)/(100)) \times 17.42 = 9.51$ g phosphate.

6. Using Equation A2.4, there are $(9.51)/(95) = 0.10$ moles of phosphate in 100 mL.

7. 0.10 moles phosphate in 100 mL is $(0.10) \times (1000) = 100$ mmol phosphate in 100 mL or $((100)/(100)) \times (10) = 10$ mmol phosphate in 10 mL of 17.42% w/v dipotassium hydrogen phosphate.

8. Using Equation A2.2, this is $(10) \times (3) = 30$ mEq of phosphate in 10 mL of 17.42% w/v dipotassium hydrogen phosphate.

References

1. Wade A, ed. *Pharmaceutical Handbook*, 19th edn. London: Pharmaceutical Press, 1980: 270.

2. Department of Health. *British Pharmacopoeia 2001*, vol. 1. London: The Stationery Office, 2001.

3. Department of Health. *British Pharmacopoeia 2001*, vol. 1. London: The Stationery Office, 2001: 271.

Appendix 3

Micronutrient preparations

Introduction

All intravenous nutrition (IVN) prescribers need to know the types of micronutrient products that can be used (if available). Some will be more

Table A3.1 Examples of available vitamin products suitable for routine micro-nutrient provision in intravenous nutrition*

Vitamin	BAPEN guidelines per 24 hours[†]	Cernevit (1 vial)[‡]	Solivito N (1 vial)[§]	Vitlipid Adult (10 mL)[§]
A	1000 micrograms	1050 micrograms (3500 IU)		990 micrograms (3300 IU)
D	5 micrograms	220 units		5 micrograms (200 IU)
E	10 mg	10.2 mg		9.1 mg
K	150 micrograms			150 micrograms
B$_1$ (thiamine)	3 mg	3.51 mg	3.1 mg	
B$_2$ (riboflavin)	3.6 mg	4.14 mg	4.9 mg	
B$_6$ (pyridoxine)	4 mg	4.53 mg	4.9 mg	
Niacin	40 mg		40 mg	
B$_{12}$	5 micrograms	6 micrograms	5 micrograms	
Folate	400 micrograms	414 micrograms	400 micrograms	
Biotin	60 micrograms	69 micrograms	60 micrograms	
C	100 mg	125 mg	113 mg	
Panthenol		17.25 mg	16.5 mg	
Glycine		250 mg		
Nicotinamide		46 mg	40 mg	

* mg, milligrams; IU, international units.
† See reference (1). BAPEN, British Association for Parenteral and Enteral Nutrition.
‡ Baxter Healthcare.
§ Fresenius Kabi.

Table A3.2 Examples of available trace element products suitable for routine micronutrient provision in intravenous nutrition

Trace element	BAPEN 24-hour guidelines in micromoles*	Decan (micromoles in 40 mL)†	Additrace (micromoles in 10 mL)‡	Multitrace 2 Plus (micromoles in 5 mL)§
Iron	20	17.9	20	
Zinc	50–100	153	100	200
Manganese	5	3.64	5	
Copper	5–20	7.55	20	
Chromium	0.2–0.4	0.29	0.2	
Selenium	0.4–0.8	0.89	0.4	0.8
Molybdenum	0.4	0.26	0.2	
Fluoride	50	76.3	50	
Iodide	1	0.01	1	
Cobalt		0.03		

* See reference (1). BAPEN, British Association for Parenteral and Enteral Nutrition.
† Baxter Healthcare.
‡ Fresenius Kabi.
§ Torbay Pharmacy Manufacturing Unit, Devon, UK (unlicensed).

difficult to obtain than others, so you will need to consider your patient population when deciding which products to stock routinely and which to order in when required.

Potential micronutrient products

Tables A3.1 and A3.2 show some examples of micronutrient preparations that are useful in common circumstances. Note that prescribing higher than maintenance provision may be unlicensed (see Chapter 9).

One vial of Cernevit is approximately equivalent to 10 mL of Vitlipid Adult plus 1 vial of Solivito N. Note that Cernevit contains no vitamin K and may therefore be more suitable for patients requiring warfarin.

Decan 40 mL is approximately equivalent to 10 mL Additrace. Drawing up 40 mL rather than 10 mL can put an additional strain on Technical Services operators (see Chapter 15), although automation may limit this. Decan contains less manganese and less iron than Additrace, which may be an advantage during initial refeeding (see Chapter 9).

You may find that you need to supplement specific micronutrients or specific groups of micronutrients within your prescribed IVN for a

Table A3.3 Examples of micronutrient preparations suitable for use in intravenous nutrition for individual patient need*

Preparation	Micronutrient content	Typical dose for 24 hours[†]	Example availability
Ascorbic acid 500 mg/5 mL	500 mg/5 mL ascorbic acid	500 mg	Celltech Pharmaceuticals Limited, Slough, UK[‡]
Copper sulphate 5 mg/5 mL	4 micromoles or 255 micrograms/mL	20 micromoles	Torbay Pharmacy Manufacturing Unit, Devon, UK[§]
Folic acid 15 mg/mL	5 mg in 0.33 mL	5 mg	Torbay Pharmacy Manufacturing Unit, Devon, UK[§]
Hydroxocobalamin 1000 micrograms/mL	1000 micrograms/mL	1000 micrograms for 3 doses	Link Pharmaceuticals, Horsham, UK[‡]
Iron chloride 100 micrograms/mL	1.79 micromoles iron in 1 mL	Up to 10 mL	Queens Medical Centre, Nottingham, UK[§]
Pabrinex	Thiamine hydrochloride 250 mg, riboflavin phosphate sodium 4 mg, pyridoxine hydrochloride 50 mg, ascorbic acid 500 mg, nicotinamide 160 mg, anhydrous glucose 1000 mg	1 pair of ampoules once a day for 3 days (nutritional indication[§]	Link Pharmaceuticals, Horsham, UK[‡]
Sodium selenite 0.00346% w/v	0.4 micromole sodium and 0.2 micromole selenium per mL	0.4–0.8 micromole	Queens Medical Centre, Nottingham, UK[§]
Zinc sulphate 1 mmol/10 mL	100 micromoles zinc and 100 micromoles sulphate in 1 mL	100–200 micromole	Torbay Pharmacy Manufacturing Unit, Devon, UK[§]

* mg, milligrams; mL, millilitres; mmol, millimoles.
[†] Depending on individual patient and reason for need (see examples in text of Chapter 9).
[‡] Licensed.
[§] Unlicensed.

Table A3.4 Typical individual micronutrient supplementation*

Micronutrient	In IVN†	Parenterally‡	Orally§
Vitamin A	Not recommended	By intramuscular injection 100 000 units every 2–4 months[2]	Not recommended route for specific replacement
Vitamin B$_{12}$** (hydroxocobalamin)	Add 1 mg into the IVN for up to 3 doses in sequential bags or every other bag	1 mg on alternate days for 3 doses by intramuscular injection or 1 mg every 1–3 months depending on indication (see Chapter 9)	Not recommended route for specific replacement
Folic acid**	Add 5 mg/day into the IVN for 2–3 weeks	If necessary, intravenous administration in 100 mL over 4–6 hours	5 mg once a day
Vitamin C (ascorbic acid)	Add 200–1000 mg/day of ascorbic acid (usually not more than 500 mg)	200–500 mg in 100 mL 0.9% w/v sodium chloride for intravenous use. Slow infusion is recommended but protect from light to prevent significant loss of active ingredient[3]. Give over 4–12 hours	100–1000 mg ascorbic acid per day
Vitamin D	Not recommended	By intramuscular injection 300 000 units (7.5 mg) usually every 3 months	Likely to need to prescribe vitamin D with calcium preparation, for example Calcichew D3 or Calcichew D3 Forte, but always check 'type' of vitamin D required[4]
Vitamin E	Not recommended; if essential, consider the standard vitamin E content of some IVN lipids	100 mg by intramuscular injection every 2–4 months	40–50 mg of D-alpha tocopherol[5]; more may be required (e.g. 100–200 mg daily)
Zinc	Add 100–200 micromoles per day into the IVN	100–200 micromoles in 100 mL sodium chloride 0.9% given over 4–8 hours	Give three times a day, for example 1 Zincomed capsule or 1 Solvazinc tablet three times a day

Table A3.4 Continued*

Micronutrient	In IVN†	Parenterally‡	Orally§
Selenium	Add 0.4–0.8 micromoles per day into the IVN	0.4–0.8 micromoles per day added to 100 mL 0.9% w/v sodium chloride and given intravenously over 12 hours	May need to consider the use of a multivitamin and trace element preparation. Consider using the injection, 0.4–0.8 micromoles per day diluted with water for injection – use immediately. May be possible to obtain an extemporaneously prepared oral solution from pharmacy
Copper	Add 10–20 micromoles per day into the IVN	10–20 micromoles in 100 mL 0.9% w/v sodium chloride for intravenous use given over 4–12 hours	May need to consider the use of a multivitamin and trace element preparation. Consider using the injection, 10–20 micromoles per day diluted with water for injection – use immediately
Others	Consider individually	Cernevit and Solivito N are compatible in 0.9% w/v sodium chloride or 5% w/v glucose[6]. Administer over 4–6 hours protected from light. Pabrinex should be given quickly after preparation[6]	Always use a complete multivitamin and trace element preparation unless contraindicated or you are correcting a specific deficiency

IVN, intravenous nutrition.

* May be unlicensed. Doses and/or frequency may need adjusting depending on the individual patient, circumstances and product availability.

† Always check stability before prescribing (see Appendix 1).

‡ If unable to add to the IVN and supplementation is required parenterally.

§ If oral/enteral administration is likely to be effective in the individual patient.

** *Caution* if giving vitamin B_{12} or folic acid without the other (see Chapter 9).

patient (see Chapter 9). Table A3.3 shows some examples of possible options that may be obtained (current in 2006). The addition of such additives to any IVN regimen may be unlicensed.

Typical specific micronutrient supplementation

Table A3.4 shows typical doses for micronutrient supplementation when adding to the IVN regimen or giving separately, either parenterally or orally. See the notes in Chapter 9 about the interpretation of reported results before giving.

References

1. Pennington C, ed. *Current Perspectives on Parenteral Nutrition in Adults: A Report by a Working Party of the British Association for Parenteral and Enteral Nutrition*. Maidenhead: British Association for Parenteral and Enteral Nutrition, 1996: 40–41.
2. Sweetman S, ed. *Martindale: The Complete Drug Reference*, 33rd edn. London: Pharmaceutical Press, 2002: 1383.
3. Trissel L, ed. *Handbook on Injectable Drugs*, 13th edition. Bethseda: American Society of Health-System Pharmacists, 2005: 154–159.
4. Sweetman S, ed. *Martindale: The Complete Drug Reference*, 33rd edn. London: Pharmaceutical Press, 2002: 1392.
5. Sweetman S, ed. *Martindale: The Complete Drug Reference*, 33rd edn. London: Pharmaceutical Press, 2002: 1394–1395.
6. British Medical Association and Royal Pharmaceutical Society of Great Britain. *British National Formulary*. London: Pharmaceutical Press, 2005: 786.

Appendix 4

High-sodium drinks and feeds for short-bowel syndrome

Introduction

Drinking around a litre a day of a high-sodium-with-glucose solution is used to limit sodium losses and to promote fluid absorption and reabsorption in patients with short-bowel syndrome (see Chapter 10). Liquids containing approximately 45 mmol glucose and 120 mmol sodium per litre have been shown to be most efficacious[1], but should only be used where other options to reduce stool losses are inadequate since they can be unpleasant to drink. Some patients self-intubate nasogastric tubes for administration or ultimately have gastrostomy tubes for long-term use.

Formulae examples for high-sodium-with-glucose powders to be made into a solution with water

Box A4.1 shows examples of possible high-sodium-with-glucose formulas for short-bowel patients.

High-sodium-with-glucose powder calculations

The high-sodium-with-glucose powder formulae in Box A4.1 can be shown to provide the stated approximate quantity.

Formula 1

The components making up formula 1 are sodium chloride BP 3.5 g, sodium bicarbonate BP 2.5 g and glucose BP 20 g.

1. Sodium chloride BP has no water of crystallisation[2] and the sodium and chloride have the same oxidation numbers (Table A2.1, Appendix 2). This means that, using Equation A2.4 and Table A2.3 from Appendix 2, the number of moles of sodium in 3.5 g of

---

Box A4.1 High-sodium-with-glucose solution formulae for patients with short-bowel syndrome

Formula 1

Components
Sodium chloride BP 3.5 g
Sodium bicarbonate BP 2.5 g
Glucose BP 20 g

Made up to 1000 mL with sterile (for jejunal administration) or potable water

Provides (approximately):
90 mmol/L sodium
101 mmol/L glucose

or

Formula 2

Components
Sodium chloride BP 2.92 g
Sodium citrate BP 4.9 g
Glucose BP 7.93 g

Made up to 1000 mL with sterile or potable water (sterile if jejunal administration)

Provides (approximately):
100 mmol/L of sodium
40 mmol/L glucose

Note: in both cases, it is the concentration that is important, not the amount

---

sodium chloride BP is $3.5/(23 + 35.5) = 0.060$ moles or, using Equation A2.1 from Appendix 2, $0.060 \times 1000 = 60$ mmol sodium (and 60 mmol chloride).

2. Sodium bicarbonate BP has no water of crystallisation[3] with a formula of $NaHCO_3$ and the sodium and bicarbonate have the same oxidation numbers (Table A2.1, Appendix 2). This means that, using Equation A2.4 and Table A2.3 from Appendix 2, the number of moles of sodium in 2.5 g of sodium bicarbonate BP is $2.5/(23 + 1 + 12 + 16 + 16 + 16) = 0.030$ moles or, using Equation A2.1 from Appendix 2, $0.030 \times 1000 = 30$ mmol sodium (and 30 mmol bicarbonate).

3. Adding up the sodium provision from both the sodium chloride and sodium bicarbonate components gives a total of $60 + 30$ mmol $= 90$ mmol.

4. Glucose BP has one water of crystallisation[4] with a formula of $C_6H_{12}O_6.H_2O$. Using Table A2.3 from Appendix 2, the proportion of glucose in glucose monohydrate is $100 \times (((6 \times 12)+(12 \times 1)+(6 \times 16))/((6 \times 12)+(12 \times 1)+(6 \times 16)+(2 \times 1)+(16))) = 100 \times (180/198) = 90.9\%$. Therefore in 20 g of glucose monohydrate the amount of glucose is $(90.9/100) \times 20 = 18.18$ g. Using Equation A2.4 and Table A2.3 from Appendix 2, the number of moles of glucose only is therefore $18.18/180 = 0.101$ moles or, using Equation A2.1 from Appendix 2, 101 mmol.

Formula 2

The components making up formula 2 are sodium chloride BP 2.92 g, sodium citrate BP 4.9 g and glucose BP 7.93 g.

1. Sodium chloride BP has no water of crystallisation[2] and the sodium and chloride have the same oxidation numbers (Table A2.1). This means that, using Equation A2.4 and Table A2.3, the number of moles of sodium in 2.92 g of sodium chloride BP is $2.92/(23+35.5) = 0.050$ moles or, using Equation A2.1 from Appendix 2, $0.050 \times 1000 = 50$ mmol sodium.

2. Sodium citrate BP has two water molecules of crystallisation as well as three sodium atoms in the molecule[5], which has a formula of $C_6H_5Na_3O_7.2H_2O$. Using Table A2.3 in Appendix 2, the proportion of sodium in the molecule is $100 \times ((23 \times 3)/((12 \times 6)+(5 \times 1)+(23 \times 3)+(16 \times 7)+(4 \times 1)+(2 \times 16)) = 100 \times (69/294) = 23.5\%$. This means that the number of grams of sodium in 4.9 g sodium citrate BP is $(23.5/100) \times 4.9 = 1.152$ g sodium. Using Equation A2.4 and Table A2.3 from Appendix 2, the number of moles of sodium only is therefore $1.152/23 = 0.050$ moles, which is $0.050 \times 1000 = 50$ mmol using Equation A2.1 (Appendix 2).

3. The total sodium content from the sodium chloride BP 2.92 g plus the sodium citrate BP 4.9 g is therefore $50 + 50 = 100$ mmol.

4. Glucose BP has one water of crystallisation[4] with a formula of $C_6H_{12}O_6.H_2O$. Using Table A2.3 in Appendix 2, the proportion of glucose in glucose monohydrate is $100 \times (((6 \times 12)+(12 \times 1)+(6 \times 16))/((6 \times 12)+(12 \times 1)+(6 \times 16)+(2 \times 1)+(16))) = 100 \times (180/198) = 90.9\%$. Therefore in 7.93 g of glucose monohydrate the amount of glucose is $(90.9/100) \times 7.93 = 7.208$ g. Using Equation A2.4 and Table A2.3 from Appendix 2, the number of moles of glucose only is therefore $7.208/180 = 0.040$ moles or, using Equation A2.1 from Appendix 2, 40 mmol.

Box A4.2 Calculating the sodium to add to an oral or enteral feed for patients with borderline short-bowel syndrome

Sodium in 1000 mL of enteral feed (mmol) + sodium
addition to 100 mL of enteral feed (mmol) = 100–120 mmol sodium per litre
(Eqn A4.1)

Volume of sodium chloride injection required (mh) =
Required sodium addition (mmol) ÷
Concentration of sodium chloride injection (mmol/mL)   (Eqn A4.2)

Adding sodium to enteral feeds

Patients with short-bowel syndrome may gain benefits in terms of sodium and fluid retention from the addition of sodium to oral or enteral feeds to create a total concentration of 100–120 mmol/L. This can be achieved by making an addition of sodium chloride injection (e.g. 30% w/v) to the feed to give the required overall concentration (Box A4.2). The aim is to ensure a round figure for the required volume of injection,

---

Box A4.3 Addition of sodium chloride injection to an oral or enteral feed

Quantity of injection to add to the feed
Using Equations A4.1 and A4.2 (from Box A4.2)

Method of addition to the feed
Check you are using the correct injection and the correct concentration for your calculations

Draw up the required volume of the injection into a syringe, using a filter needle if the injection is presented in a glass ampoule

Discard the needle if using a filter needle

Add the injection solution to the container of enteral feed (avoid using a needle because of the safety risk but, if absolutely necessary, replace needle first)

Ensure adequate mixing to avoid pooling of the addition

Discard enteral feed container according to local infection control policy or after a maximum of 24 hours if leaving in the original container or 4 hours if the feed is decanted into another container

Note: use strict aseptic technique throughout

which gives a final concentration of between 100 and 120 mmol sodium per litre in as simple and practical a way as possible. The calculations will vary depending on the concentration of sodium chloride injection used. For example, 30% w/v sodium chloride provides 5.13 mmol sodium per mL, but lower concentrations provide less sodium per unit volume.

These additions should be made as safely as possibly and, if drawing up from a glass ampoule, the injection solution should be filtered before it is added to the feed to prevent shards of glass being administered (Box A4.3).

References

1.   Nightingale J, Lennard-Jones J, Walker E, Farthing M. Oral salt supplements for jejunostomy losses: comparison of sodium chloride capsules, glucose electrolyte solution, and glucose polymer electrolyte solution. *Gut* 1992; 33: 759–761.
2.   Department of Health. *British Pharmacopoeia 2001*, vol. 1. London: The Stationery Office, 2001: 1481–1482.
3.   Department of Health. *British Pharmacopoeia 2001*, vol. 1. London: The Stationery Office, 2001: 1473–1474.
4.   Department of Health. *British Pharmacopoeia 2001*, vol. 1. London: The Stationery Office, 2001: 803.
5.   Department of Health. *British Pharmacopoeia 2001*, vol. 1. London: The Stationery Office, 2001: 1482–1483.

Index

accuracy, nutrition regimens 235
acid instillations 190
Addiphos 273
Additrace 282
administration rates 116, 165–6
administration routes 55–7, 61
adult intravenous formula calculation
    form 171
airflow, clean-rooms 265
alanine transferase (ALT) 209
albumin 111
alcohol 128, 189, 190
allergies 60
ALT *see* alanine transferase
amino acids 82–6, 195
anorexia nervosa 4
antibiotics 55, 183–4
antimotility drugs 158
arrival *see* delivery of bags
ascorbic acid 129, 132, 283
aseptic technique 248–9, 263–4, 266
aspartate transferase (AST) 209
aspiration 15–16
AST *see* aspartate transferase
atomic masses 275
audit 217

bags
    cold chain 269
    precompounded 161–3, 173, 243
    prescribing 238
    standardisation 240
    starting 246–50
    technical services 233–44
    triple-chamber 161–6, 243, 264
    ward procedures 245–53
balance *see* electrolyte balance; fluid
    balance
basal metabolic rate (BMR) 76, 77
best-prescribed routes 55, 57
biliary obstruction 197
biochemistry

electrolyte prescribing 121–3
IVN eligibility 44–5
monitoring 207
sodium levels 105
spurious abnormalities 98–9, 102
biotin deficiency 135
blockages *see* occlusion
blood glucose monitoring 208
BMI *see* Body Mass Index
BMR *see* basal metabolic rate
Body Mass Index (BMI) 37–8, 225
body weight 37–8, 46, 76
bone 111, 112, 211
British Association for Parenteral and
    Enteral Nutrition (BAPEN) 213–14
B vitamins 130–1, 133–4, 135

cabinet airflow patterns 265
calcium
    jejunostomy patients 158
    monitoring 202
    prescribing considerations 110–13
    refeeding syndrome 103–5
    renal disease 149
    replacement values 119, 120
carbohydrates 195–6, 208
cardiac failure 154
cardiorespiratory status 47
catheter-related sepsis (CRS) 54, 182–4
catheters 28–31, 179–81, 185–9
central venous catheters (CVC) 28–9, 190
Cernevit 282, 285
chemical contaminants 236
chemical pathology/biochemistry 221
chemical stability 234, 259–60
chest X-rays 181
chronic malnutrition 38
clean rooms 264–7
clinical examination of patient 45–8
clinical history 35–51
clinical records 65–7, 217
clinical review 210–11

clinical trials 33
cold chain 267–9
colloid fluids 72
'complete' oral nutritional supplements 8
complications 2, 13–18, 32, 179–200, 228
component stocks 242–3
compounding 233–45, 268
compromise, regimens 174–8
computer-generated intravenous nutrition
    prescription charts 176
concentrations 192, 273–6
consent 4
containers 260
contamination 235, 264–5
    see also aseptic technique
continuing IVN stability 87–8
contract services 173, 240–3
cool packs 269
copper 137, 285
copper sulphate 283
costs 174, 230–1, 242
CRS see catheter-related sepsis
crystalloid fluids 72, 74

data collection forms 224–8
data management 217, 223–4
Data Protection Act 223
deficiencies 125–37, 140–3
delivery of bags 173, 245, 267–9
deposition, occlusive 185
descriptive bag names 163
DEXA see dual-spectrum X-ray
    densitometry
diarrhoea, ETF-related 16–17, 54–5
diet 7, 38, 126–7
dietitians 218
disease-specific feeds 9
displaced ETF tubes 15
documentation
    data collection forms 171, 224–8
    IVN decisions 65–9
    IVN prescriptions 175, 178
    nutrition regimens 235–6
Doppler vein imaging 179
drugs
    administration routes 55–7
    concurrent fluids administration 263
    electrolyte effects 98
    ETF administration problems 58–9
    ETF diarrhoea 17
    gastrointestinal tolerance 54–7
    IVN regimens 262–3
    IVN routes/interactions 53–61, 109,
        185, 186, 191
    micronutrient depletion effects 128
    monitoring 203, 206–7

dual-spectrum X-ray densitometry
    (DEXA) 211
duration of administration 192
duration of contract 242

education of practitioners 217, 230
efficacy of IVN 32–3
elderly patients 141
electrolyte balance 95–123
    biochemistry results interpretation 98–9
    deficits 117
    emergency precompounded IVN 251
    excessive fluid loss 96–7
    homeostatic mechanisms 95–8
    imbalance consequences 102
    IVN bags 164–6, 240, 246, 247
    IVN contracting 243
    IVN–drug regimes 60
    metabolic complications 196–7
    monitoring 202, 209
    practical issues 121–3
    refeeding syndrome 102–5
    regimen compromise 174
    renal handling 97
    restricted electrolytes 169
    salts 258, 274
    specific severe abnormalities 118–21
    standard prescribing 115–17
    unplanned stops on IVN 253
    urinary electrolytes 100–1
    ward prescribing 167
elemental oral feeds 9
emergency situation 63, 239, 249–50
endorsement, prescription charts 68–9
energy requirements
    estimations 75–8
    glucose 79–80
    lipids 81–2
    liver disease 151
    nitrogen sources 82–3
    recommended amounts 78–83
    regimens 164
    renal disease 149–50
enforcement of IVN 4
enteral tube feeding (ETF)
    before/after major surgery 26
    combined with IVN 32
    complications 13–18
    drug administration problems 58–9
    drug-related diarrhoea 54–5
    feed types 12–13
    IVN comparison in postop period 27
    prescription records 67–8
    prescription review before IVN 50–1
    problems requiring IVN 19
    recent nutrient intake history 38–9

sodium 290
sodium chloride 290–1
starting IVN bags 247
tube types 10–12
essential fatty acids 81
estimated requirements 75–8, 84–5
ETF *see* enteral tube feeding
ethical issues 4–5
expiry, compounded products 244

failed IV placement 247, 252
fatty acids 82
feeding rate 16, 116, 251
feeds 8–9, 12–13, 16–17
fibre-containing oral feeds 9
fibrin clots 187–8
fibrinolytic occlusion clearance 190
filtration, IVN 193–4
final bag release 236–8
fine-bore peripheral venous catheters 30
fish oil-based lipids 90
fluid balance
    cardiac failure 154
    concurrent drug administration 263
    excessive loss 96–7
    IVN bags 246
    IVN complications 195
    liver disease 150–1
    monitoring 203, 205–6
    osmolality 73–4
    overload/oedema 73
    pre-IVN status 47
    renal disease 148–9
    requirements 71–83
    restriction 169
    review before IVN 48–50
    sodium biochemistry 100
    starting IVN bags 247
    type of fluid to give 72–3
    unplanned stops on IVN 253
    volume needs estimation 72
folate 130–1, 135
folic acid 283
food fortification 7–8
food intake records 50
forms 171, 224–8
formulations of drugs 58, 59
funding 230–1, 239

gastric pooling 16
gastric tubes 11
gastrointestinal tract
    examination 47–8
    fistulae 155–6
    function 14, 15–17, 21, 39–43, 54–5
    monitoring 201, 203–4

gastrostomy tubes 12, 14, 15
general examination, pre-IVN 45–7
general status, monitoring 201, 203
glucose
    energy provision 79–80
    energy source advantages 85
    IVN formulations 75
    monitoring 202
    regimen stability 172
glucose-to-lipid energy ratios 86
glutamine 90–2, 167
glyceryl trinitrate 193
grams 275–6
guidelines *see* National Institute for
        Clinical Excellence
guidewires, GI tract perforation 13

haematology 43–4, 207–8
haemoglobin 43–4
hair 46
hand-written prescription charts 176
HEPA filters 265
'heparin' locking 188
hepatobiliary surgery 22
high jejunal fistulae 156–9
high-output gastrointestinal fistulae
        155–6
high-sodium drinks 287–91
high-sodium-with-glucose drinks 288
history
    clinical 35–51
    gastrointestinal function 39–43
    major organ function 42–3
    nutrient intake 37–9
homeostatic mechanisms 95–8
home patient workload 216–17
homocysteine 130–1
hospital admission 1, 7
hydrocortisone 193
hydroxycobalamin 283
hypoalbuminaemia 17, 19
hypoglycaemia 25, 251
hypotonic fluids 157–8

ileocolic anastomosis patients 159–60
ileostomy anastomosis patients 159–60
ileus, postoperative 40, 41
independent prescribing 220–1, 238
indications
    enteral tube feeding 10
    intravenous nutrition 19–28
    nutrition support 3–4
infection 17, 54, 201, 203
    see also sepsis
inflammatory markers 44, 208
infusates interaction 53–61, 109, 186

infusion duration 262
infusion rate 240
in-line filtration 193–4, 258
inpatient workload 216
INR *see* international normalised ratio
insulin 80, 153, 262
insulin-resistance 195–6
integrity of bags 247
intensive care units 121
interactions 53–61, 109, 185, 186, 191
internal lumen sepsis 184
international normalised ratio (INR) 202
intestinal function 14, 15–17, 39–43,
    54–5
intrahepatic cholestasis 198
intravenous access 28–31, 48, 252–3
intravenous catheters 179–81, 183, 247
intravenous drugs *see* drugs
intravenous fluid charts 49–50, 175
intravenous nutrition (IVN)
    cardiac failure 154
    clinical examination/history 35–51
    complications 32
    contracting 240–3
    decision-making 63–9
    drug routes/interactions 53–61, 109,
        186
    electrolytes 95–123
    ETF comparison post operation 27
    ethical/legal issues 4–5
    fluid balance requirements 71–83
    indications 19–28
    jejunostomy 156–9
    liver disease 150–2
    micronutrients 125–44
    overview 19–33
    pancreatitis 152–3
    prescription charts 53–61
    regimen stability 260–3
    renal compromise regimens 147–50
    respiratory failure 154–5
    short bowel syndrome 155–60
    specialised macronutrients 89–92
    starting 86–7
    stopping 250–3
    surgical patients 21–8
    Technical Services 233–6
    timing 245–6
iron chloride 283
iron deficiency 136
IVN *see* intravenous nutrition

jejunal tubes 11
jejunocolic anastomosis patients 159
jejunostomy 156–9
tubes 12, 14, 15

kilocalories (kcal) 75

laboratory monitoring 207
    fluid balance 203, 205–6
    general status 201, 202, 203
    glucose 202, 208
    long-term IVN patients 211
    nutrition support eligibility 43–5
lactase deficiency 17
leaks in bags 238
legal aspects 4–5
licensing Technical Services 243–4
light, chemical stability 260
lines *see* catheters
linoleic acid 81, 82
linolenic acid 81, 82
lipids
    central line occlusion 191
    energy provision 81–2
    energy source advantages 85
    metabolic complications 196
    regimens 170
    specialised 89–90
    stability 259, 261
liver disease 21, 150–2
liver function 197–9, 202, 209–10
logistics 222, 241
long-chain triglycerides 91
long-term patients 27–8, 38, 210–11
lumen use 29

macronutrients
    balancing provision 85–6
    components for regimens 173–4
    intravenous nutrition contracting 242
    ratios in regimens 169
    requirements 83–92
    specialised 89–92
magnesium
    jejunostomy patients 158
    prescribing considerations 109–10
    refeeding syndrome 103–5
    renal disease 149
    stability of IVN regimens 261
    suggested replacement values 120
    typical replacement values 119
major organ function 42–3
malabsorption 127
malnutrition 1–2, 38
manganese deficiency 137
manufacturers' licences (UK) 243–4
market contracts 242
measurement units 273–6
mechanical obstruction 185, 191
medical patients 1, 38, 53–5, 127
medicine charts 175

Medicines and Healthcare Products
    Regulatory Agency (MHRA) 244
medium chain triglycerides 89, 91
metabolism
    see also basal metabolic rate; resting
      metabolic rate
    abnormalities 203
    BMR adjustments to stresses 77
    ETF complications 14, 17–18
    IVN complications 195–9
metastatic calcification 113
MHRA *see* Medicines and Healthcare
    Products Regulatory Agency
microbiology
    IVN eligibility 45
    monitoring 207
    stability of IVN regimens 234–5, 263–9
micronutrients 125–44, 281–91
    additions to regimens 167
    depletion 46, 126–37
    elderly patients 141
    emergency pre-compounded IVN 251
    increased initial provision 139–40
    IVN contracting 243
    liver disease 152
    metabolic complications 197
    monitoring 137–8, 210
    NICE recommendations 125–6
    prescriptions 138–44
    regimen compromise 174
    role in the body 131
    specific supplementation 144
    unbalanced provision 129
    wound healing 142
microparticulate risks 193–4
milliequivalents 275–6
millimoles 275
monitoring
    clean rooms 266–7
    electrolytes 101–2, 116–17
    fluid balance 203, 205–6
    general status 201, 202, 203
    IVN 201–32
    micronutrient status 137–8, 202, 210
    nutrient intake 203, 204–5
    nutrition lines 206
    renal function 209
mouth signs 46
multiple electrolyte sources 97–8
MUST (Malnutrition Universal Screening
    Tool) 225

nails 46
names, nutrition bags 163
nasogastric tubes 11, 13–14
nasojejunal tubes 12, 13–14

National Institute for Clinical Excellence
    (NICE) recommendations 201, 213
    energy provision 78–9
    indications for nutritional support 27,
      63
    micronutrients 125–6
    nutrition support guidelines 3
    post-operative ETF 25, 27
    refeeding problems 118
nausea, ETF-related 16
neurological aspects 21, 48
NICE *see* National Institute for Clinical
    Excellence
nicotinic acid (vitamin B$_3$) 134
nitrogen
    emergency pre-compounded IVN 251
    non-energy uses 83–6
    pre-compounded/sterilised triple-
      chamber bags 164
    regimen stability 172
    requirements calculation 75, 84–5
    sources 82–3, 90–2
non-energy uses of nitrogen 83–6
non-nitrogen energy-to-nitrogen ratio 86
non-steroidal anti-inflammatory drugs
    (NSAIDs) 193
non-viable contaminants 236
NSAIDs *see* non-steroidal anti-
    inflammatory drugs
NST *see* nutrition support teams
nutrient intake 37–9, 50–1, 203, 204–5
nutritional status 45–7
nutritional supplements *see* oral
    nutritional supplements
nutrition support teams (NSTs) 36, 69,
    213–17, 255
nutrition teaching 219

obesity 76
occlusion 15, 58, 185–9, 190
octreotide 158
oedema 73
oesophageal problems 21
off-site delivery 269
olive oil-based lipids 89–90, 91
operator assessment (clean rooms) 266
oral diet 41, 247
oral medicines tolerance 55
oral nutritional supplements 7–10, 59,
    67–8, 138–9
ordering frequency 173
organic salts 258, 273
orogastric tubes 11
osmolality 73–4, 81
overfeeding problems 77–8
oxidation numbers 271–2

oxygen 260

Pabrinex 283
packaging 269
pancreatic disease 22, 152–3
patient comfort 245
patient details 36–7
patient numbers 173
patient reviews 66–7
patient workload 216–17
percentage calculations 275–6
perioperative period 25
peripheral catheters 29–31
peripherally inserted central catheters
     (PICC) 29–30
peripheral vein feeding regimens 164
peripheral vein thrombophlebitis (PVT)
     189–90, 191–4
peripheral vein thrombosis 252
pharmaceutical calculations 276–80
pharmacological incompatibilities 53–61,
     109, 185, 186, 191
pharmaconutrient oral feeds 9
phosphate
     prescribing considerations 113–15
     refeeding syndrome 103–5
     renal disease 149
     replacement values 119, 120
     salts 273
physical stability 234, 257
physiological stress 77, 95–6
PICC see peripherally inserted central
     catheters
plasma levels
     albumin 111
     electrolytes 98–100, 101–2, 103–5
     glucose 208
     micronutrients 142–3
     potassium 107–9
platelets 44
polymeric complete oral supplements
     8–9
polymeric fat-free oral supplements 9
poor oral intake 20
portal bacterial translocation 197
positive pressure airflow 265
postinsertion ETF tube-related problems
     14–15
postoperative period 25–7, 40, 41
postrenal impairment 147
potassium phosphate 272
potassium requirements
     cardiac failure 154
     prescribing considerations 107–9
     refeeding syndrome 103–5
     renal disease 148

suggested oral/enteral replacement
     values 120
typical replacement values 119
practice journals 220
precipitation 257–8
pre-compounded bags 161–3, 173, 243
predigested oral feeds 9
pre-existing GI disease 39
preoperative period 24–5, 26
prerenal impairment 147
prescription charts 176–8
     allergies 60
     drug routes/interactions 53–61
     endorsing 68–9
     intravenous fluids 49–50
     nutritional supplements 59
     review 53
     specialist 60–1
prescriptions 255
     see also regimens
     bag release 238
     checking when starting IVN bags 247
     documentation 175
     electrolytes 105–17, 121–3
     enteral feeding 50–1
     location for regimens 178
     micronutrients 138–44
     nutrition support team 220–1
     patients with specific problems 147–60
product ranges 8–9, 89–91, 161–3, 241
prophylaxis 184, 188–9, 192–4
protein requirements 83–6, 149–50,
     151–2
purchasing contracts 242
pyridoxine (vitamin B_6) 135

randomised controlled trials (RCTs) 33
rates of administration 116, 251
RCTs see randomised controlled trials
rebound hypoglycaemia 25
recent gastrointestinal history 39–42
recent nutrient intake 38–9
recommencement of IVN 88–9
recommended energy provision see
     National Institute for Clinical
     Excellence
refeeding syndrome
     electrolyte balance 102–5
     emergency intravenous nutrition 250
     fluid balance 73, 78
     risk criteria 104, 117–18, 141
     starting IVN cautiously 86–7
     Wernicke–Korsakoff syndrome 128
referrals 36–7
reflux with ETF 15–16
refrigeration 268

regimens
  calcium provision 112–13
  compromise 174–8
  contracts with suppliers 173
  electrolytes 115–17
  fluid component 75
  glucose-to-lipid energy ratios
    calculation 86
  macronutrient components 173–4
  magnesium provision 109–10
  micronutrient prescriptions 138–44
  phosphate provision 114–15
  potassium provision 108
  prescribing location 178
  selection 161–78
  sodium provision 106
  specific problems 147–60
  stability 170, 233–5
  technical services 233–6
release delays 268
renal function 97, 101, 209
renal impairment 114, 122, 147–50
respiratory failure 154–5
resting metabolic rate (RMR) 76
results unavailability 121–2
reviews 48–51, 53, 66–7, 210–11
riboflavin (vitamin B$_2$) 134
risk factors 104, 117–18, 141, 192–4
RMR *see* resting metabolic rate
role overlap 217–21

salts 157, 258, 271–80
  see also electrolytes
SBS *see* short-bowel syndrome
Schofield equations 76
scurvy 129, 132
seasonal factors 269
section 10 exemption (unlicensed) (UK)
  243
Seldinger technique 30, 179–81
selenium 137, 285
sepsis
  catheter-related 255
  intravenous catheters 247
  IVN catheters 183
  liver function 197
  signs 182
  unplanned stops in IVN 252
serum *see* plasma
short bowel syndrome (SBS) 155–60,
  287–91
short-term IVN 42, 64
SIADH *see* syndrome of inappropriate
  antidiuretic hormone secretion
skin 46
small intestinal disease 22–3

small vein diameter 192
sodium bicarbonate 190
sodium chloride 157, 258, 290–1
sodium requirements
  calculation for high-sodium drinks 290
  cardiac failure 154
  enteral feeds 290
  fluid balance 100
  liver disease 150–1
  prescribing considerations 105–7
  refeeding syndrome 103–5
  renal disease 148
sodium selenite 283
solubility in alkaline conditions 191
specialised preparations 9, 89–92, 169
specialist advice 216
specialist nutrition nurses 218
specialist prescription charts 60–1
specials licence (UK) 243
specific micronutrients 144
specific vitamin supplementation 140–3
stability 257–70
  chemical 234, 259–60
  continuing IVN 87–8
  drugs added to IVN regimens 262
  electrolyte additions 166
  IVN electrolytes 117
  IVN regimens 170–2, 260–3
  lipids 259, 261
  physical 234, 257
standardisation of bags 240
standard prescribing 115–17, 261–2
starting IVN 139–40, 246–50
starvation 95–6
steatosis 197–8
steering committees 214
sterilisation 264
sterilised triple-chamber bags 161–2
stock flexibility 173
stopping IVN 250–3
storage space 173
strategic model 214–15
stress factors 77, 95–6
structured medium-chain lipids 89
subcutaneous ports 31
supervisory model 214–15
supplementary prescribing (UK) 144,
  220–1, 238
supplements *see* oral nutritional
  supplements
support services 241, 245
surfaces, clean 264–5
surgical patients 1, 2, 21–8, 40, 41, 247
swallowing difficulties 20–1
syndrome of inappropriate antidiuretic
  hormone secretion (SIADH) 106

teaching 219, 220
technical services 221, 233–44
temperature, chemical stability 260
tenders for IVN supplies 241
thiamine (vitamin B$_1$) 133–4
thrombophlebitis 189–94
thrombosis 185, 191
timing aspects 245–6, 269
    see also duration
tolerance, drugs 55–7
'top-slicing' funding model 230–1
toxicity effects 132–7
trace elements 202, 210, 260, 282
training 217, 230
triglycerides 82, 89
triple-chamber bags 161–6, 243, 264
Trissel (book) 263
tube insertion problems 13–14
tube types, ETF 10–12
tunnelled cuffed catheters 31

UK *National Diet and Nutrition Survey*
    126
unbalanced micronutrient provision 129
units of measurement 273–6
unplanned stops 252–3
urinary electrolytes 100–1
ursodeoxycholic acid 199

vascuports 31
venous access 28–31, 48, 252–3
venous irritability 192
viable contaminants 236
visual bag inspection 238
vitamins 129–37
    see also micronutrients
    A deficiency/toxicity 132
    B$_1$ deficiency/toxicity 133–4
    B$_2$ deficiency/toxicity 134
    B$_3$ deficiency/toxicity 134

B$_6$ deficiency/toxicity 135
B$_{12}$ deficiency/toxicity 135
C deficiency/toxicity 129, 132, 283
D deficiency/toxicity 133
E deficiency/toxicity 133
K deficiency/toxicity 135
monitoring 202
poor storage/processing/production
    127–8
specific deficiencies 132–7
stability of intravenous nutrition
    regimens 261
volume approximations 167–8
vomiting 40

wards
    clinicians 221
    nurses 221
    pharmacists 221
    prescribing 167
    procedures 245–54
    rounds 219
warfarin 197
warming bags 248
waste reduction 240
WBC *see* white blood cell
weather effects 269
weight *see* body weight
Wernicke–Korsakoff syndrome 128
white blood cell (WBC) count 44
withdrawal of IVN 5
withholding of IVN 5
workflows 245–6
workloads 216, 222, 238–9
wound healing 142

X-rays 181

zinc 136, 284
zinc sulphate 283